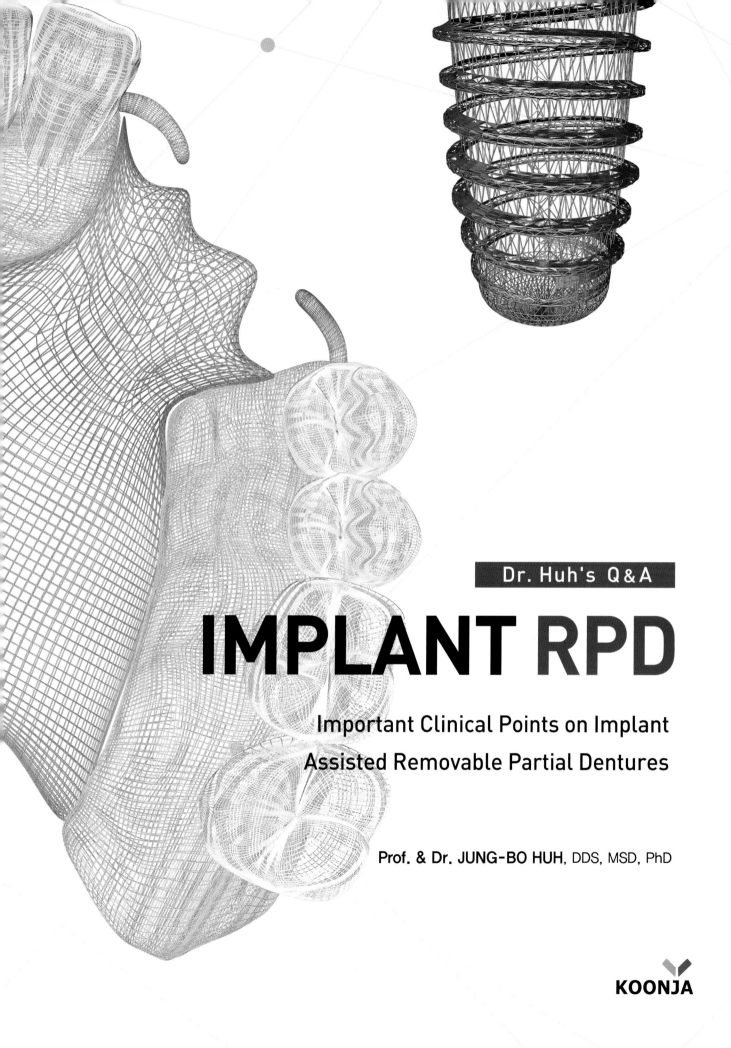

# IMPLANT RPD

Important Clinical Points on Implant
Assisted Removable Partial Dentures

Prof. & Dr. JUNG-BO HUH, DDS, MSD, PhD

KOONJA

Dr. Huh's Q&A

# IMPLANT RPD

1st Print : 2021-06-04
1st Publication : 2021-06-21

Autho : Jung-bo Huh
Editor : Su-in Han, Kyung-eun Lee
Text Designer : Ran-hee Yang
Cover Designer : Jae-wook Kim
Illustrator : Eun-bin Bae, Hakyoung Yu

Permissions may be sought at Koonja's rights department:
Tel : (82)-31-943-1888
Fax : (82)-31-955-9545
www.koonja.co.kr

Printed in South Korea
First Edition, © 2021 Koonja publishing, Inc.

ISBN 979-11-5955-717-0

# IMPLANT RPD

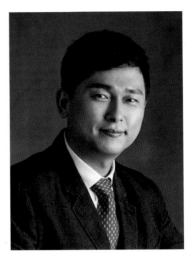

Prof. & Dr.
**JUNG-BO HUH**

Dr. Huh graduated from the School of Dentistry, Pusan National University, Korea in 2002. He finished the Residency program for the specialty of Prosthodontics at the Ajou University Hospital and received his Ph.D. degree at the School of Dentistry, Yonsei University, Korea in 2011. Dr. Huh is Professor of Prosthodontics at the School of Dentistry, Pusan National University. He has published over 140 scientific papers and ten books in the field of dentistry. He has lectured extensively on dental implants and prosthodontics. Dr. Huh is also the Head of the Department of Prosthodontics, Pusan National University Dental Hospital. Dr. Huh has been honored with the "Student Research Fellowship Award" by the IADR Implantology Research Group in 2009, "IADR Hatton Award" by IADR Korean Division in 2010, and "Young Scientist Award" by the Korean Academy of Prosthodontics in 2012. Recently, he was honored as the grand prize winner of the "Yeon-Song Dentistry Prize" the most famous award in the field of Korean dentistry in 2018. Dr. Huh also has over 25 patents to his name and he is CEO of the company PNUADD which develops advanced dental devices based on his novel ideas.

It was definitely not a simple decision. Quite frankly, I was hesitant about whether it was appropriate for me to discuss implant-assisted removable partial dentures (IARPD) despite the contradictory advice from many experts that - in addition to my own lack of clinical experience - there is sparse scientific evidence on the discipline itself.

Working at a university hospital, I was exposed to a significant number of returning patients bearing problems from previous treatments. One of the common findings in patients treated with IARPD was that clinicians tended to rely too much on implants. There are several arguments related to the extent of protection implants require; nevertheless, there is no doubt that implants are vulnerable to lateral and rotational forces rather than vertical.

I would not say that IARPD is a new treatment method at all. When only a few natural teeth remain to be used as abutment teeth, implants augment the retention, support, and stability of the RPD. One of the basic principles of RPD, as we have learned in school, is to avoid exerting adverse forces on abutment teeth. I believe that abiding by this principle when treating IARPD would reduce any potentially harmful forces on implants.

There have been many clinical and laboratory trials in published literature research papers research papers on implant overdentures and relatively numerous established treatment methods, whereas there is almost nothing available on IARPD. However, the argument I would like to pose concerns the conceptual difference between implant overdentures and IARPD. What is the difference between the concepts underlying the treatments of IARPD and conventional RPD? I believe that these three types of treatments are all based on the same principles.

IARPD is not specifically difficult to understand, but having a thorough understanding of the basic principles of conventional RPD and its complicated intraoral movements can be challenging. Over the past ten years, I have been giving numerous lectures nationwide, and I have aggregated numerous questions from the audience.

This book is a compilation of answers to those questions and the thoughts that I have mulled over while studying IARPD. Most of the clinicians asked for solutions for problems encountered in their clinical cases. It was difficult to give definite answers to their questions without fully understanding the various conditions of their specific clinical cases. Hence, I resolved to provide problem-solving skills rather than giving a definite answer.

This book contains topics that aim to briefly summarize the basic principles of RPD. Details such as diagnostic procedures in RPD patients, components of RPD such as major and minor connectors, and laboratory procedures were omitted. I have tried to provide the readers with a better understanding of how to efficiently distribute forces and control denture movements to minimize adverse stress on implants. Therefore, I would recommend this book to those who have the basic knowledge of the principles of RPD; otherwise, reference to an RPD textbook is strongly recommended.

I, sincerely and humbly, hope that this book will strengthen your understanding of IARPD rather than provide a rigid go-to solution. And I hope that it could ultimately provide your patients with a solution that will enable them to pursue a better treatment option.

June, 2021

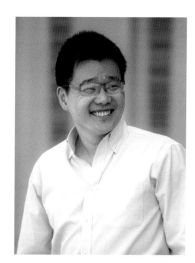

Prof. & Dr.
**TAE KIM**

Biography

Dr. Tae Kim is Chair of the Removable Prosthodontics Section in the Division of Restorative Science, Herman Ostrow School of Dentistry, University of Southern California, (USC), Los Angeles, California, US.

Dr. Kim is a recipient of multiple grants, patents and, awards in digital removable prostheses, implant research, and biomaterials, and gives lectures on the international platform on CAD/CAM dentures. Dr. Kim focuses on digital removable prostheses and education using the latest technologies.

He has authored a lecture series in Removable Prosthodontics and the Prosthodontics Review Book at Herman Ostrow School of Dentistry of USC and is also the author of numerous clinical and research articles in CAD/CAM dentures and implant dentistry.

He completed postgraduate training in Prosthodontics at the Herman Ostrow School of Dentistry at USC and obtained his Doctorate of Dental Science from the Seoul National University, South Korea.

It is with tremendous pleasure that I write the foreword to Dr. Huh's book which describes the science of removable partial prosthodontics taking implant therapy to a new level both clinically and academically, and has been a best-seller in Korea.

Dr. Huh spent a year as a visiting scholar in the Herman Ostrow School of Dentistry at the University of Southern California (USC), Los Angeles, California, USA., where many of his thoughts and experiences described in this book were heavily discussed, debated and redefined.

In this book, the clinicians will discover the basics of implant therapy in conjunction with removable partial denture, design considerations and modification, and multiple case studies done at the Prosthodontics Department, Pusan National University.

The concepts presented in this book have been taught at the Pusan National University of Education, South Korea, and help students and residents to learn various modifications through implant therapy with partial denture. The goal of the author is to refresh classic knowledge of partial denture design and implants, then briefly discuss different clinical approaches tested in his clinic at the Pusan National University and to share the outcome with clinicians in other countries.

I hope this book will receive wide attention from the practice of removable prosthodontics, and that therefore both clinicians and their patients will benefit from it.

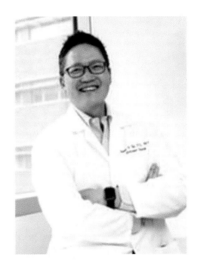

Prof. & Dr.
**Reuben Kim**

Dr. Reuben Kim is Professor and Chair in the Section of Restorative Dentistry, Division of Constitutive and Regenerative Sciences, at the University of California Los Angeles (UCLA) School of Dentistry.

Dr. Kim received both DDS and PhD from UCLA and joined the UCLA School of Dentistry as a faculty in 2006. Since then, he has been heavily involved in teaching in many capacities including the course chair for the Direct Restorations, the course chair for the Treatment Planning Clinic, director of the Restorative Advanced Clinical Training (ACT) program, and director of Research Collaborative Program. He practices general dentistry in the UCLA Faculty Group Dental Practice.

Dr. Kim has more than 70 publications, over 110 abstracts, and over 40 invited lectures. Through his research programs, he has mentored close to 100 individuals, including post-doctoral fellows, visiting scholars, and PhD/MS/DDS/undergraduate students. Dr. Kim's research focuses on investigating the underlying mechanisms of regenerative and reparative pulp biology, medication-related osteonecrosis of the jaw (MRONJ), and craniofacial bone biology. His research projects have been funded by numerous agencies including R01s from NIH/NIDCR.

Being in a teaching institution close to 20 years, I encountered numerous patients who have only few natural teeth left – situations where we as clinicians start thinking how they can be better served by providing affordable, economical, but yet ever-lasting dental treatments. This is more so with a significant increase in implant utilizations in elderly individuals in the clinics nowadays. In this book, Dr. Huh truly address this well by introducing the concept of IARPD that are more patient-centric.

This book not to explain the fundamentals of RPD, but also goes above and beyond to apply the current knowledge to IARPD. IARPD can be quite beneficial by boosting up both retention and support to the RPD; however, the concept of IAPRD may remain controversial. Through many years of clinical experiences as well as modifications from the heated debates and arguments, Dr. Huh really put them all together well in this book in a reader-friendly manner to understand fundamental principles of IARPD and to avoid potential pitfalls.

I'd like to congratulate Dr. Huh for publishing this important and timely addressed concepts in implant-assisted removable partial denture (IARPD). It is my hope that this book can challenge many educators and practitioners to another level of practicing dentistry.

# Contents

CHAPTER 5

# Representative clinical researches and the summary derived from those studies on IARPD with implant surveyed prostheses

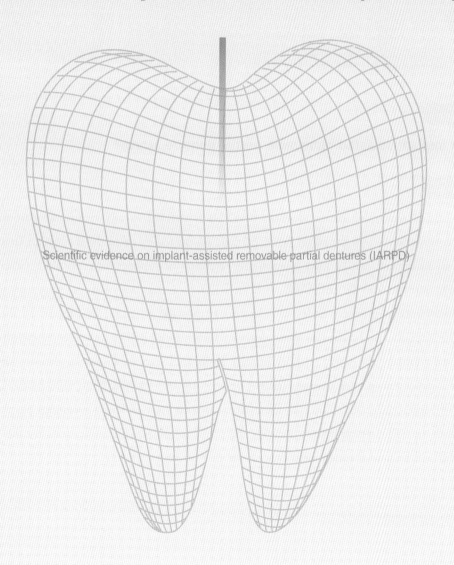

CHAPTER
# 1

# Scientific evidence on implant-assisted removable partial dentures (IARPD)

Scientific evidence on implant-assisted removable partial dentures (IARPD)

*Chapter 1.*

# Scientific evidence on implant-assisted removable partial dentures (IARPD)

Scientific evidence on implant-assisted removable partial dentures (IARPD)

## Question

**What is an implant-assisted removable partial denture (IARPD)?**

## Answer

An implant-assisted removable partial denture (IARPD) is defined as any removable partial dental prosthesis that covers and rests on dental implants, partially supported by them. In general, an attachment of the denture to an implant can be used for attaining retention or support for edentulous patients.

In an IARPD, implants can be combined with an RPD in a number of ways. They can be used with healing abutments or precisely fitting attachments to provide retention or support to the RPD. Alternatively, the implants can be used as abutments for conventional RPDs, or telescopic crown RPDs.

In international journals, the terms such as implant-supported removable partial denture (ISRPD), implant-retained removable partial denture (IRRPD), and implant-assisted removable partial denture (IARPD) are used interchangeably. However, these terms actually have different meanings based on the role of implants in the RPD, which is quite complex and prone to subjective classification. For this reason, the term IARPD will be used throughout this book for ease of understanding.

**Question**

## What are the advantages and disadvantages of IARPDs over conventional RPDs?

**Answer**

### Advantages of IARPDs

(1) The use of implants under distal extension denture bases can provide occlusal support.

- It is easier to chew with the molar part and develop stable chewing habits.

(2) Tooth and tissue-supported RPDs can be changed to tooth (implant)-supported RPDs which results in increased support and reduced movement of the denture.

- The reduced denture movement can enhance mastication. As a result, the harmful stress on the residual teeth would be reduced.

(3) Denture base area can be properly adjusted, resulting in a better fit and greater comfort.

- Patients will experience less extension of denture base, less discomfort, and adapt to the dentures more easily.

(4) Aesthetics

- Because of its attachment to implants, the IARPD does not require many direct retainers such as clasps. This helps the patients to have a more aesthetic outcome.

### Disadvantages of IARPDs

(1) Surgical and economic burden

- Although only a few implants are used, implant placement requires surgery, and its cost may be burdensome to some patients.

(2) Complicated denture fabrication

- It is very difficult to balance the three movements that may occur under pressure in IARPDs: extensive movement of the edentulous mucosa, physiological movement of the natural teeth, and the rare movement of the implants.

(3) Side effects such as peri-implant bone loss or denture fracture

- Increased support from additional implants can raise the risk of fracture of denture components due to concentrated stress around the implants or weakened denture parts.

## What has been the problem with conventional RPDs?

It is important to understand both the advantages and disadvantages of conventional RPDs. In conventional distal extension RPDs, occlusal forces are distributed through the residual ridges, reducing the stress on the remaining teeth. However, the abutment teeth are prone to plaque accumulation, and the lateral forces acting on the residual teeth may cause secondary caries and periodontal disease. The factors influencing the prognosis of conventional RPDs have been studied in several clinical trials. The results of some of these studies have been summarized below.

### (1) Causes of loss of abutment teeth

In the early years of usage, several disadvantages of conventional RPDs were reported in scientific literature. Carlsson et al.(1976) reported that caries developed in 93% of the observed cases after 4 years of RPD delivery. In addition, 15% of the abutment teeth experienced increased mobility after a year of RPD delivery. They also reported that 23% and 60% of the patients stopped using their dentures for various reasons after 4 and 13 years, respectively. During the time of the Waerhaug study (1968), the overwhelming consensus was that conventional RPDs were harmful to the oral cavity, and they were therefore not recommended. In this study, it was determined that RPDs were transitional dentures used during the transition to complete dentures. In other words, these studies suggested that despite the clear advantages of RPDs, such as occlusal function recovery and aesthetic improvement, their harmful effects on the residual ridge and abutment teeth could not be overlooked.

On the other hand, Rudd et al.(1996) reported that precise guiding planes on abutment teeth were helpful in preventing mobility and periodontal disease of the abutment teeth of RPDs. Subsequently, Derry et al.(1970) and Bergman et al.(1971) reported that there was no destruction of the periodontal tissue after RPD delivery. The clinical observations of patients with RPDs showed neither an increase in the mobility of the abutment teeth nor deterioration of the gingival index.

What could have yielded the positive outcomes, unlike the unfavourable results reported earlier? Lundqvist (1967) assessed the factors influencing the prognosis of RPDs leading to the loss of abutment teeth. The study showed that the factors related to the loss of teeth were influenced by independent factors, including RPDs, caries, and periodontal disease. Therefore, any harmful forces exerted by the RPD potentially resulting in teeth loss should be corrected immediately following delivery. If this is not done, acceleration of abutment teeth loss will be inevitable due to the combined effects of mechanical stress and plaque deposition by the components of the RPDs.

Recently fabricated RPDs have better prognosis because oral care, including periodontal treatment of residual teeth, has to be well maintained prior to RPD delivery. Maeda et al.(1980) reported that plaque accumulation on abutment teeth increased with denture delivery. However, with proper tooth brushing, the plaque accumulation scores markedly decreased.

### (2) RPD design to preserve abutment teeth

Becker et al.(1994) listed six basic principles of designing an ideal RPD which can preserve the abutment teeth.

<u>**Basic principles of designing an RPD by Becker et al.(1994)**</u>

1) A rigid major connector should be included.
2) The appropriate placement of rests can effectively distribute occlusal forces.
3) Mesial rests are effective for distal extension RPDs.
4) Guiding planes are effective in retaining and stabilizing the RPD.
5) RPI clasps with I-bars are recommended for direct retainers of distal extension RPDs.
6) Altered casts help to stabilize and increase support in RPDs.

Previously, there was a non-rigid support concept that resolved the difference in pressure displacement between the abutment teeth and the soft tissue with a stress-breaker designs, but a series of studies have proven that the concept is not valid.

The rigid support theory emphasizes the need for a strong connection between the abutment teeth and the RPD, which in turn demands strong support from the abutment teeth and utilizes soft tissue support to the maximum. As a result, the abutment teeth and denture base can suppress the movement of the RPD. In other words, a properly designed RPD has appropriate rests, retainers, connectors, and the correct base, which will minimize RPD movement and evenly distribute occlusal forces throughout the abutment teeth and the soft tissue of the edentulous areas. Therefore, based on previous studies, it can be concluded that properly designed RPDs do not damage abutment teeth, but rather protect them.

### (3) Advantages of using implants for distal extension RPDs

The use of posterior implants for distal extension RPDs increases the possibility of suppressing the tissue-ward movements of the distal extension area by providing support, whether from the use of implant

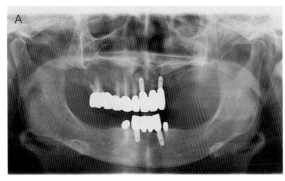 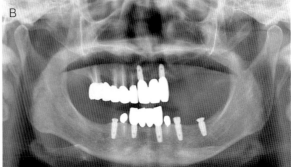

**Figure 1.** In cases in which the distal extension area is broad, additional implants can be used to extend the supportive area.

surveyed crowns, attachments, or healing abutments. In other words, tooth-tissue supported RPDs can be changed to tooth supported RPDs by using implants.

Figure 1 shows a 60-year-old female patient who had implants inserted without the need for bone grafts to increase support, stability, and retention of her existing RPD.

In the case of a patient having few anterior teeth as shown in Figure 1A, the tissue-ward movement of the distal extension area is increased, and the increase of lateral forces exerted by the direct retainers located around the anterior abutment teeth can result in excessive, harmful stress. In particular, the inappropriate placement of indirect retainers can increase RPD movement. If additional implants are placed in the posterior area as shown in Figure 1B, the firm support area increases, and the tissue-ward movement of the RPD is prevented. As such, if the movement of the RPD and the lateral force transmitted to the abutments are reduced, the RPD will be more comfortable and last longer.

Attachments can be used to provide support and retention with additional implants. In this case, if the path of RPD insertion determined by the surveyed crown is similar to that of the attachment as shown in Figure 2, the attachment will survive longer, and the amount of lateral force delivered to the implant fixture will be reduced. This will be explained in more detail in later chapters. Therefore, it is recommended that the path of RPD insertion should be considered at the time of implant placement. The obvious method is to use a surgical guide stent as shown in Figure 2, which allows you to set the approximate path of RPD insertion digitally and design the implant surgical guide stent in that direction.

As shown in Figure 3, the implants were inserted during a flapless surgery using a surgical guide stent designed to position the implants in a direction similar to the path of RPD insertion. Two implants were inserted in the premolar area to obtain both retention and support using attachments. The implant in

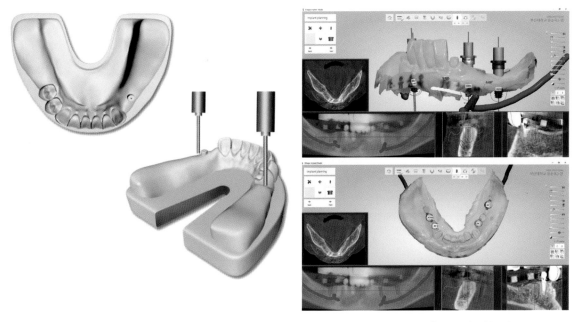

**Figure 2.** In the case of using implant attachments, a surgical guide stent can be manufactured taking into account the path of RPD insertion and path of attachment.

the left second molar area was designed to provide support only by a healing abutment. All the implants contributed to enhanced stability. With the clasp of the existing RPD removed, the remaining denture base, with its tissue support, can be reduced in size. In this case, however, a fracture of the RPD itself may occur, which would require adjustments. A more detailed description will follow in the chapters to come.

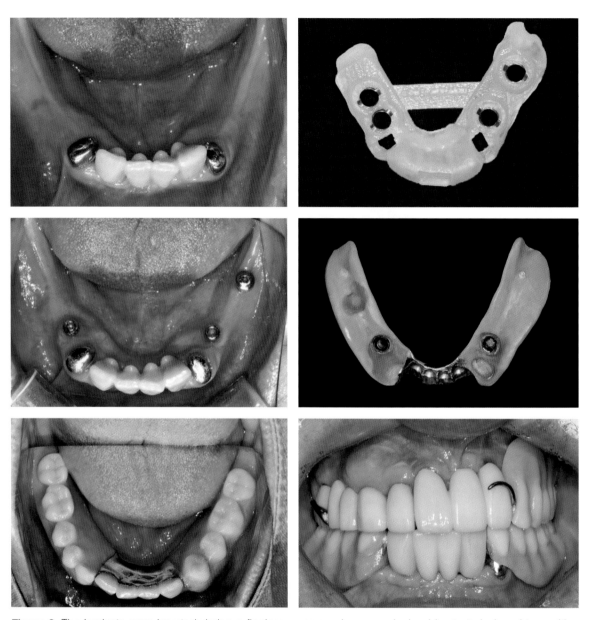

**Figure 3.** The implants were inserted during a flapless surgery using a surgical guide stent designed to position the implants in a direction similar to the path of RPD insertion. Two implants were inserted in the premolar area to simultaneously obtain retention and support using the attachments. The implant in the left second molar area was designed to provide support by a healing abutment. All these implants contributed to the stability of the denture.

**Differences in the existing literature surrounding implant overdentures and IARPDs**

**Answer**

Based on existing literature, two consensus statements (McGill, 2002 and York, 2009) suggested that the first choice of prosthetic treatment for edentulous patients was an overdenture with two implants placed in the mandible (2-IOD). In other words, the 2-IOD is a treatment with high patient satisfaction and has become the global standard for prosthetic treatment of edentulous patients. On the other hand, current research surrounding IARPD is insufficient compared to that of overdentures, and most of the published articles about IARPD are case reports. Controversial aspects related to IARPDs will be discussed in Chapter 3.

In clinical applications, the mandibular 2-IOD can be a reliable treatment method. Though IARPDs lack empirical evidences, the use of implants under the denture base of RPDs in clinical situations has been shown to reduce their movements and provide reliable occlusal support. Therefore, IARPDs can be considered to be a promising treatment for future clinical applications. It is important that clinicians have full knowledge of the advantages and disadvantages of IARPDs, and make sure they are sufficiently explained to patients.

**Question**

**How do the roles of implants differ with regards to support, stability, and retention between implant overdentures and IARPDs?**

**Answer**

When treating edentulous cases, clinicians often encounter patients with severe alveolar bone loss. Treating these patients with IODs can be challenging, particularly because the insertion of implants in the molar area proves difficult. Therefore, in such cases, implants are usually placed in the anterior region.

The role of implants in 2-IODs is to prevent dislodgement, consequently reducing the tissue-away movement of the dentures. This indicates that the implants are establishing the retention of the dentures (see Chapter 2). With the masticatory force transmitted to the implants, there is an element of additional support. Excessive support, however, may eventually create an unstable denture as the patient may become reliant on chewing with the anterior part of the denture where the implants were placed. It is preferable to utilize the retentive element of the attachment when the denture is about to the presence of dislodgement.

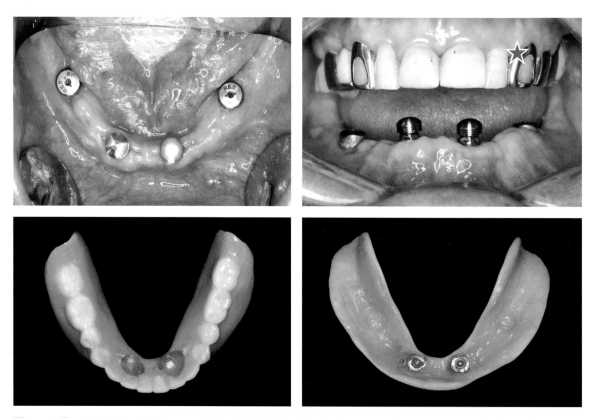

**Figure 4.** Four-implant-assisted removable partial denture. The ball type attachments were used only on the anterior implants for retention and healing abutments were used on the posterior implants for support.

★ This fixed prosthesis was fabricated about 20 years ago, but the patient did not want to change to a new prosthesis.

Figure 4 shows an example of another edentulous patient. In this case, it was possible to place implants in the molar areas as there was sufficient amount of alveolar bone structure. Therefore, a total of four implants were placed: two in the anterior, and two in the molar region. The ball type attachments were used only on the anterior implants for retention; healing abutments were used on the posterior implants for support. Implants at all corners of the trapezoid contributed to enhancing retention and vertical occlusal support. The attachments and the healing abutments at the four corners eliminated almost all denture movements.

For 2-IODs (Implant retained overdenture), the two implants may provide retention only; however, by placing two additional implants into the molar areas, the IOD will have both retention and support. This type of denture is called a 4-IOD, an implant-supported overdenture.

The terms referring to implant combined removable partial dentures can be confusing. The term implant-retained removable partial denture (IRRPD) can be used if retention is mainly supplied by the implants. It may also be called an implant-supported removable partial denture (ISRPD) if the implants mainly serve to support the denture. In this textbook, the term implant-assisted removable partial denture, (IARPD) will be used to include both concepts.

Whether the implants are used mainly to support or to retain the denture, the location of the implants as well as the types of attachments to be used will be determined. If a single implant is placed below the denture base to prevent the movement of a distal extension RPD, the implant mainly acts as a supporting factor. Figure 4 shows advantageous implantation sites and the types of attachments that can provide proper retention and support.

The 2-IOD often uses implants mainly to obtain retention of the denture. In IARPDs they are often used to obtain not only retention, but also support or stability of the RPDs.

## Question

### What does the literature have to say about IARPDs?

## Answer

There have been many studies about fixed prostheses using implants, and the empirical support for this treatment is evident. In terms of implant overdentures, the scientific evidence is well established, and more research is being actively conducted. However, the scientific evidence for the success of IARPDs is still limited. In addition, studies on IARPDs are not yet specific enough, and it is clear that there are limitations to the existing literature. The reason is that, unlike fixed prostheses and complete dentures, IARPDs involve natural teeth, implants, and soft tissue, altogether resulting in numerous treatment methods with countless variables. Moreover, it is very difficult to make a standardized experimental model and apply effective variables in clinical studies. In 2015, Chatzivsileiou K et al. reviewed the research on IARPDs in order to centralize the data in one place. An electronic search was conducted on the PubMed database for published english-language articles that contained information about implant-assisted RPDs. A review of these articles indicated that combining dental implants with RPDs created a cost-efficient prosthetic protocol that can combat the problematic aspects of treatments using an RPD alone. However, it also mentioned that more well-designed studies are still needed to provide robust information about critical issues, such as design guidelines, long-term survival rates of implants associated RPDs, and their effect on patients' quality of life (see Chapter 5).

Treatment methods using IARPDs are not significantly different from those of conventional RPDs.

Finally, it is a thorough understanding of the basic concepts of RPDs that will eventually aid in the devlopment of effective treatments with IARPDs. Additionally, it is crucial to understand the characteristics of implants, so that they can be placed in the right location minimizing the lateral forces exerted on the implant, thereby improving long-term prognosis. All things considered, IARPDs may become one of the most effective treatment methods.

Table 1. Summary table of the literature on IARPDs, including treatment guidelines and clinical results.

| Clinical researches | | | | |
|---|---|---|---|---|
| Authors | Implant survival rate | Complication and maintenance | Patient satisfaction | Implant location |
| Bortolini et al.(2011) | • 93.75% survival rate<br>• 8 years follow up<br>• 32 patients, 64 implants | • Implant<br>– Biologic: 4 implant loss (in 4 patients)<br>– Technical: 2 abutment screw loosening (in 2 patients)<br>• Tooth<br>– Biologic: 29 tooth loss<br>• Denture<br>– Relining: 93 (in 32 patients)<br>– Tooth substitution: 29 (in 24 patients)<br>– Resilient cap replacement: 1 per year (in all patients) | • 5-point questionnaire (on a scale from 1 to 5)<br>• from 1.31±0.43 to 4.59±0.47 | • Mx: (n=42)<br>– Lateral incisor: 1<br>– Canine: 21<br>– First premolar: 14<br>– Second premolar: 6<br>• Mn: (n=22)<br>– Canine: 10<br>– First premolar: 9<br>– Second premolar: 3 |
| Mijiritsky et al.(2005) | • 100% survival rate<br>• 2-7 years follow up<br>• 15 patients, 33 implants | • 1 Rupture<br>• No clinical signs (mobility or gingival inflammation around implants) | ND | ND |
| Mitrani et al.(2003) | • 93.8% survival rate<br>• 1-4 years follow up<br>• 10 patients, 16 implants | • Implant<br>① only vertical stops:<br>– Biologic: 1 implant loss<br>– Technical: 2 screw loosening, 1 framework fracture, 2 pitting of the healing abutment surface<br>② retention elements:<br>– Biologic: 1 mucosal hyperplasia (in 1 patient)<br>• Prosthetic complication<br>① only vertical stops: 1 framework fracture, 2 pitting of healing abutment surface | • 5-point questionnaire (on a scale from 1 to 5)<br>• from 1.2 to 5 | ① only vertical stops: Mx (n=8), Mn (n=1)<br>② retention elements: Mx (n=3), Mn (n=4) |
| Grossmann et al.(2009) | • 97.1% survival rate<br>• 9 months to 10 years follow up<br>• 35 patients, 67 implants | ND | ND | • Mx: (n=28)<br>– Anterior: 9<br>– Premolar: 13<br>– Posterior: 6<br>• Mn: (n=39)<br>– Anterior: 18<br>– Premolar: 5<br>– Posterior: 16 |

| | | | | |
|---|---|---|---|---|
| Kaufmann et al.(2009) | • 93.8% survival rate<br>• 1-8 years follow up<br>• 60 patients, 93 implants | • Implant<br>– Biologic: 3 implant loss (before loading), 3 implant loss (after loading), 8 peri-implantitis (in 7 patients), 1 mucosal hyperplasis (in 1 patient)<br>– Technical: 12 abutment screw loosening 4 wear of abutment<br>• Tooth<br>– Biologic: 3 tooth loss (root coping), 8 caries, 3 periodontitis, 2 gingival hyperplasia<br>– Technical: 21 recementation of root coping; 1 wear of ball anchor<br>• Prosthetic complication<br>– Implant: 10 matrix loosening, 38 matrix tightening, 22 matrix replacement<br>– Tooth: 4 matrix loosening, 45 matrix tightening, 41 matrix replacement<br>– Denture:<br>– Repairs: 3 fracture of resin denture base<br>– Adjustments: 6 redesign of existing denture, 24 sore spots, 15 relining of denture, 28 occlusal adjustment, 2 excessive prosthetic tooth wear | ND | • 1–2 implants placed per denture<br>• Mx implants + abutment teeth:<br>– Lin (2 abutments): 3<br>– Tri (3 abutments): 8<br>– Quad (4 abutments): 34<br>• Positions of Mx implants :<br>– Central incisor: 4<br>– Lateral incisor: 5<br>– Canine: 18<br>– First premolar: 23<br>– Second premolar: 18<br>• abutment teeth:<br>– Lin (2 abutments): 12<br>– Tri (3 abutments): 5<br>– Quad (4 abutments): 3<br>• Positions of Mn implants:<br>– Central incisor: 1<br>– Lateral incisor: 1<br>– Canine: 13<br>– First premolar: 10<br>– Second premolar: 2 |
| Krennmair et al.(2007) | • 100% survival rate<br>• 38 months<br>• 22 patients, 60 implants | • Implant<br>– Technical: 3 screw loosening<br>• Tooth<br>– Technical: 3 tooth fracture<br>• prosthesis: 4 adjustment | ND | • Mx implants (1–5 per patient):<br>– Lateral incisor: 8<br>– Canine: 19<br>– First premolar: 10<br>– Second premolar: 14<br>– First molar: 9<br>• Mx abutment teeth:<br>– Central incisor: 4<br>– Lateral incisor: 6<br>– Canine: 13<br>– First premolar: 5<br>– Second premolar: 7<br>– First molar: 7<br>– Second molar: 1 |

| | | | | |
|---|---|---|---|---|
| Mijitsky et al.(2007) | • 100% survival rate<br>• 5 years follow-up<br>• 21 patients | ND | ND | ND |
| Payne et al.(2017) | • After 3 year: 100% survival rate<br>• After 10 year: 91.7%(6 implants in 5 patients)<br>• 10 years follow up<br>• 36 patients, 72 implants | • Implant<br>– Biological: 6 implant loss in 5 patients<br>• Tooth<br>– Biological: 1 abutment tooth loss, 2 all anterior teeth | ND | • Implant: Bilateral first or second molar region, 1 implant per side<br>• Abutment teeth: Bilateral first premolar or canine, one clasp per side |
| Rinke et al.(2015) | • 100% survival rate, 95.8% success rate<br>• 5.84 ¡¾ 3 years (3.0-12.2y)<br>• 14 patients, 24 implants | • Implant<br>– Biologic: 5 implants with mucositis (in 3 patients), 1 implant with peri-implantitis (in 1 patient)<br>– Technical: 5 abutment screw loosening<br>• Tooth<br>– Technical: 4 tooth loss (crown fracture) | ND | • Mn:<br>– 2 second incisor<br>– 12 first premolar<br>– 3 second premolar |
| Bemhart et al.(2012) | • 2 years follow up<br>• IARPD group: 100% survival rate: 16 patients, 40 implants<br>• IRO group: 97.6% survival rate: 19 Patients, 84 implants | • IARPD group<br>– Technical: 1 abutment screw loosening<br>• IRO group<br>– Technical: 2 abutment screw loosening<br>– Biologic: 2 implant loss, 2 peri-implantitis | ND | • IARPD group: Mx (n=14), Mn (n=2)<br>– Quad (4 abutments): 5<br>– Poly (5-9 abutments): 11<br>• IRO group: Mx (n=12), Mn (n=7)<br>– Tri (3 abutments): 1<br>– Quad (4 abutments): 14<br>– Poly (5-6 abutments): 3 |
| Grossmann et al.(2008) | • 95.5% survival rate<br>• Mean 31.5 months follow up<br>• 23 patients, 44 implants | • Implant<br>– Biologic: 2 implant loss (in 1 patient) | • Reported Improvement in:<br>– Masticatory efficacy (87%)<br>– Esthetics (78%)<br>• IARPD rating:<br>– Very comfortable (65%)<br>– Comfortable (22%)<br>– Uncomfortable (13%) | • Mx:<br>– Lateral incisor: 1<br>– Canine: 8<br>– First premolar: 10<br>– Second premolar: 1<br>– First molar: 1<br>– First molar: 5<br>• Mn:<br>– Central incisor: 1<br>– 12 lateral incisor: 12<br>– 5 canine: 5 |

| | | | | |
|---|---|---|---|---|
| Hug et al.(2006) | • 2 years follow up<br>• IARPD group: 100% survival rate: 14 patients, 20 implants<br>• IRO (implant-retained overdenture) group: 98.2% survival rate: 15 Patients, 57 implants | <IARPD group><br>• Implant: 5 matrix loosening, 6 matrix tightening<br>• Tooth<br>– Technical: 1 tooth loss, 2 recementation of root coping<br>– prosthetic: 2 matrix loosening, 7 matrix tightening<br>• Prosthesis: 2 repair, 8 adjustment<br><br><IRO group><br>• Implant<br>– Biologic: 1 implant loss,<br>– Technical: 9 abutment loosening<br>– prosthetic: 1 matrix loosening, 2 matrix tightening<br>• Prosthesis: 5 repair, 15 adjustment | • IRO group was more satisfied compared to IARPD group in: Comfort of wear, Stability of prosthesis<br>• IRO group was more satisfied compared to OvP (only-tooth–supported overdenture) group in: (only-tooth–supported overdenture) General satisfaction, Speaking ability, Comfort of wear, Stability of prosthesis, General problems | • IARPD group: Mx 10, Mn 10<br>• IRO group: Mx 33, Mn 24 |
| Bae et al.(2017) | • 100% survival rate<br>• IARPD (implant attachment combined RPD) group: 23.5 months follow up: 12 patients, 28 implants<br>• ISBRPD (implant surveyed bridge combined RPD) group: 26.7 months follow up: 10 patients, 25 implants | • IARPD group: 64% Locator male replacement, 22% denture repair<br>• ISBRPD group: 67% Denture relining, 33% Denture repair | ND | ND |
| Oh YK et al (2020) | • 100% survival rate<br>• 24 patients, 80 implants<br>• average 27.6 months follow up<br>• All cases are IARPDs with implant surveyed prostheses | • Denture related complications : 2 clasp fractures, 1 rest fracture<br>• Implant surveyed prosthesis-related complications: 1 decementation, 1 severe marginal bone resorption, 1 porcelain fracture | ND | • Mx: incisor 4, canine 6, premolar 21, molar 13<br>• Mn: incisor 8, canine 12, premolar 15, molar 1<br>• Based on considerations of RPD abutment symmetry, implants were placed in positions of occlusal contact with opposing natural or implant teeth |

| | | | |
|---|---|---|---|
| Kang SH et al (2020) | • The survival rate of total 58 implants was 93.1%: 95.1% for implants supporting surveyed crowns and 88.2% for implants used in overdentures<br><br>• 21 patients, 58 implants<br><br>• average 47.9 months follow up | • Complications in overdenture IARPDs were 1.8-folds higher than that of surveyed crown IARPDs<br><br>• In surveyed crown IARPDs: 31.2% of the complications were related to crowns<br><br>• In overdenture IARPDs: 45.8% were related to tissue, and 37.5% to denture<br><br>• 70% of the total implants showed marginal bone loss less than 1.5 mm.<br><br>• The marginal bone loss was higher in Kennedy class I than in Kennedy class III | ND |
| | | | • Limited information<br><br>• Anterior:13, Posterior:28<br><br>• Mx :22 Mn: 19<br><br>• According to Kennedy classification<br>  - I :10<br>  - II : 18<br>  - III : 3<br>  - IV : 10 |

| Guidelines for implant placement | | | |
|---|---|---|---|
| authors | purpose | models | results |
| Cunha et al.(2008) | Evaluation of the best implant location by means of, the bi-dimensional finite element method, through stress distribution and support structure displacement of a distal extension RPD (DERPD) associated with an implant. | • 5 mandibular models<br>– Model A (MA)–represented a mandibular hemi-arch without posterior abutment, with the presence of #33 only<br>– Model B (MB)–similar to MA, presenting a conventional DERPD with a distal plate in the proximal region of #33, replacing #s 34, 35, 36, and 37.<br>– Model C (MC)–similar to MB, differing from it by the presence of a 10 × .75 mm Brånemark osseointegrated implant, located in the distal cusped region of the second molar.<br>– Model D (MD)–similar to MC, differing from it by the location of the implant being in the region of the first molar median cusp.<br>– Model E (ME)–similar to MC, differing from it by the location of the implant being in the region of the second bicuspid, under the DERPD base. | • Approximating implant in direction of support teeth was benefit for stress distribution.<br><br>• Locating the implant near of the abutment tooth influenced positively the distribution of stresses on the analyzed structures.<br><br>• The presence of the implant in all positions relieved the regions with reference to the alveolar edge when compared with the model with only the DERPD.<br><br>• The closeness of the implant in the direction of the support tooth positively affected the tension distribution on the structures analyzed. |

| | | | |
|---|---|---|---|
| Verri et al.(2007) | Assessment of the influence of length and diameter of the implant incorporated under the saddle of DERPD, acting as support. | • 6 hemi-mandibular models<br>– model A; without removable partial denture<br>– model B; removable partial denture only<br>– model C; removable partial denture and implant of 3.75 × x mm<br>– model D removable partial denture and implant of 3.75 × x3 mm<br>– model E removable partial denture and implant of 5 × x mm<br>– model F removable partial denture and implant of 5 × x3 mm. | • The introduction of the implant reduced tensions, mainly at the extremities of the edentulous edge.<br>• Both the length and diameter tended to reduce tensions as their dimensions increased.<br>• The increase of the diameter of the implant had a great influence on the decrease of von Mises tension values by the methodology of this study but did not influence the displacement values.<br>• It is a sound choice to use as large an implant as possible in the association of implant and removable partial denture. |
| De Freitas Santos et al.(2011) | Evaluation of the displacement and stress distribution transmitted by a DERPD associated with an implant placed at different inclinations (0, 5, 15 and 30 degrees) in the second molar region using the two-dimensional finite element method. | • 6 hemi-mandibular models<br>– model A; only with the presence of the natural tooth 33<br>– model B; similar to model A, with the presence of a conventional DERPD replacing the missing teeth<br>– model C; similar to the previous model, with a straight implant (0 degrees) in the distal region of the ridge, under the denture base<br>– model D; similar to model C, with the implant angled at 5 degrees in the mesial direction<br>– model E; similar to model C, with the implant angled at 15 degrees in the mesial direction<br>– model F; similar to ME, with the implant angled at 30 degrees in the mesial direction. | • The use of an implant as a support decreased the displacement of alveolar mucosa for all inclinations simulated.<br>• The stress distribution transmitted by the DERPD to the supporting structures was improved by the use of straight or slightly inclined implants. |

| | | | |
|---|---|---|---|
| Pellizzer et al.(2010) | Biomechanical Behavioral Assessment of DERPD associated with an Implant and different retention system by bidimensional finite element method. | • 5 hemi-mandible models<br>– model A; hemi-mandible with a canine and a DERPD<br>– model B; hemi-mandible with a canine and implant with a healing abutment associated to a DERPD<br>– model C; hemi-mandible with a canine and implant with an ERA attachment associated to a DERPD<br>– model D; hemi-mandible with a canine and implant with an O'ring attachment associated to a DERPD<br>– model E; hemi-mandible with a canine and implant-supported prosthesis associated to a DERPD. | • It is possible to conclude that oblique loads increased the displacement and von Mises stress levels in all analyzed models.<br>• model C (with the ERA-Sterngold retention system) was the most favorable system for the association based on the stress distribution |
| Cunha et al.(2011) | Evaluation of the displacement tendency of the supporting structures of a DERPD associated to the implant with different inclinations and implant localizations through a two-dimensional finite-element method. | • 16 mandibular models | • Models with horizontal ridge exhibited the highest values in the region of the median or distal cusp of the first molar.<br>• In the ridge, the association with anterior implant decreased the tendency of displacement of the denture base and relieved the region of the ridge between the abutment tooth and the implant regarding the values.<br>• For models with distally ascending ridge, the highest values were exhibited in the region between the distal cusp of the first molar and the mesial cusp of the second molar, in all models<br>• Models with descending-ascending ridge exhibited the highest values in the region of the distal and median cusps of the first molar. |

Mx = Maxilla, Mn = Mandible, IARPD = implant-assisted removable partial denture (removable partial denture and overdenture design), OvP = overdenture prosthesis (only-tooth–supported overdenture); IRO = implant-retained overdenture (only-implant–supported overdenture), ISBRPD = implant surveyed bridge removable partial denture, DERPD = distal extension removable partial denture, ND = no data

**How are the supporting structures of teeth and implants different, and how do their movements differ?**

Unlike natural teeth, implants lack periodontal ligaments (PDLs), which act as shock absorbers in natural dentition. Also, it is scientifically proven that when a severe bending moment is applied to the alveolar bone around the implant, a fulcrum is created, leading to peri-implant bone resorption. Therefore, previous studies suggest that the success of fixed implant prostheses can be obtained by creating controlled occlusions.

Table 2. **Comparison between characteristics of teeth and implants.**

|  | Tooth | Implant |
|---|---|---|
| Connection | Periodontal Ligament (PDL) | Osseointegration<br>Functional Ankylosis |
| Proprioception | Periodontal mechanoreceptors | Osseoperception |
| Tactile sensitivity | High | Low |
| Axial mobility | 25-100 µm | 3-5 µm |
| Movement phases | Two phases<br>Primary: non-linear and complex<br>Secondary: linear and elastic | One phase<br>Linear and elastic |
| Movement patterns | Primary: immediate movement<br>Secondary: gradual movement | Gradual movement |
| Fulcrum to lateral force | Apical third of root | Crestal bone |
| Load-bearing characteristics | Shock absorbing function<br>Stress distribution | Stress concentration at crestal bone |
| Signs of overloading | PDL thickening, mobility,<br>wear facets, fremitus, pain | Screw loosening or fracture, fracture of the<br>abutment or prosthesis, bone loss, implant fracture. |

It is natural that excessive occlusal force on implants leads to peri-implant bone resorption or implant failure. However, some studies have reported that even when excessive vertical force was applied, no marginal bone resorption was observed. Therefore, marginal bone resorption may not always appear when excessive occlusal force is transmitted to the implant vertically. What is clear, however, is that when excessive lateral forces are applied due to early or heavy contact, bone loss and excessive marginal bone absorption may occur. This fact has been proven in many studies and is clearly observed in many clinical practices.

It is imperative to understand that both teeth and implants experience horizontal movement due to the elastic deformation of the bone being put under an excessive force, and the movement of teeth is larger than those of the implants. The major difference between implants and teeth is in the movement following the initial small force. In other words, teeth have periodontal ligaments, so they initially have relatively larger movements under a small load (about 500g), but implants have little to no movement.

It became clear that greater success with an IARPD would be possible if the lateral forces on the implants were minimized when designing the RPD. Many studies on implant overdentures have also suggested the use of a bilateral balanced occlusion established with a lingualized occlusion to achieve denture stability in patients with normal alveolar ridges, and a monoplane occlusion for patients with severely absorbed alveolar ridges to reduce lateral movements. A study by Peroz et al.(2003) also demonstrated that if the bilateral balanced occlusion and canine guidance are established, denture movement may be minimized. Although the details of these studies differ slightly, they all concluded that an increased success rate of implants can be achieved by minimizing the lateral forces and thus reducing the denture's lateral movements.

Schools teach how to effectively prevent the movement of RPDs and how to reduce the harmful forces acting on abutment teeth. The point is that the success of IARPDs begins with a more thorough application of the basic concepts of RPD fabrication.

Though several relevant clinical studies were presented internationally, this book will cover only two of those studies to thoroughly detail how to obtain success with IARPDs (see Chapter 5).

### Question

**What is the scope of IARPDs covered in this book?**

### Answer

In this book, the author will divide IARPDs into four different categories.

(1) After insertion of a small number of implants for partially edentulous patients, RPDs are fabricated using attachments including healing abutments.

(2) After insertion of a small number of implants for partially edentulous patients, RPDs are fabricated using implant surveyed crowns.

(3) After insertion of a small number of implants for completely or partially edentulous patients, overdenture type prostheses are fabricated using bars and attachments.

(4) After insertion of a small number of implants for completely edentulous patients, overdenture type

protheses are fabricated using attachments.

Even when there is a single implant placed in an edentulous jaw, because the implant holds the denture and limits its movements, it creates an axis of denture rotation. So, in this book, implant overdentures are treated in the same manner as RPDs. The cases of (1), (3), and (4) have more scientific evidence in comparison to the case of (2). Relevant literature will be briefly mentioned in the following chapters.

Considering the differences between implants and teeth described above, more thorough efforts should be made to control the movement of the RPD and to reduce the lateral or rotational force applied to implants. Chapters 2 and 3 describe the basic concepts of RPD design. However, detailed explanations of the basic elements of RPD, such as major and minor connectors, are not covered in this textbook. The focus will be on the design of RPD components around abutments and the overall control of RPD movements to understand how to reduce the lateral force acting on the abutments, including implant attachment and prosthesis. Please refer to other textbooks for specific details on other elements. In Chapter 4, each of the four different types of IARPDs mentioned above will be studied by analyzing each case, and specifics will be discussed.

Finally, the last chapter will present clinical studies based on the cases in which the author tries to faithfully apply the basic principles and concepts of RPDs as described in this book.

## REFERENCES

1.  Carlson GE, Hedegard B and Koivumaa KK. Syudies in partial dental prosthesis III. A longitudinal study of mandibular partial dentures with double extension saddles. Acta odont scand 1962;20:95-119.

2.  Carlsson GE, Hedegard B and Koivumaa KK. Studies in partial dental prosthesis IV. Late results of treatment with partial dentures. J oral rehabil 1976;3:267-272.

3.  Carlsson GE, Hedegard B and Koivumaa KK. Studies in partial dental prothesis II. An investigation of mandibular partial dentures with double extension saddles. Acta odont scand 1961;23:215-237.

4.  Waerhaug J. Periodontology and partial prosthesis. Int Dent J 1968;18:101-107.

5.  Rudd KD, O'leary T. Stabilizing partially weaked teeth by using guide plane removable partial denture, a preliminary report. J Proth Dent 1966;16:721-726.

6. Derry A, Ulrik B. A clinical survey of removable partial denture after two years usage. Acta Odontol Scand 1970;28:581-598.

7. Bergman B, Hugoson A, Olsson C. Periodontal and prosthetic considerations in patient treated with removable partial dentures and artificial crowns, a longitudinal two-years study. Acta Odontol Scand 1971;29:621-638.8.

8. Lundquvist C. Tooth mortality in Sweden, A statistical survey of tooth loss in the swedish population. Acta Odontol Scand 1967;25:289-322.

9. Maeda T, Kroone H, Stoltze K, Runov J, El Ghamrawy E, Brill N. Concatenation of variations in plaque formation with variations in crevicular temperature. J Oral Rehabil. 1980;7:199-203.

10. Becker CM, Kaiser DA, Goldfogel MH: Evolution of removable partial denture design. J Prosthodontics 1994;3:158-166

11. Feine JS, Carlsson GE, Awad MA, Chehade A, Duncan WJ, Gizani S, Head T, Lund JP, MacEntee M, Mericske-Stern R, Mojon P, Morais J, Naert I, Payne AG, Penrod J, Stoker GT Jr, Tawse-Smith A, Taylor TD, Thomason JM, Thomson WM, Wismeijer D. The McGill Consensus Statement on Overdentures. Montreal, Quebec, Canada. May 24-25, 2002. Int J Prosthodont 2002;15:413-414.

12. British Society for the Study of Prosthetic Dentistry. The York consensus statement on implant-supported overdentures. Eur J Prosthodont Restor Dent 2009;17:164-165.

13. Bortolini S, Natali A, Franchi M, Coggiola A, Consolo U. Implant-retained removable partial dentures: an 8-year retrospective study. Journal of Prosthodontics: Implant, Esthetic and Reconstructive Dentistry 2011;20:168-172.

14. Mijiritsky E, Ormianer Z, Klinger A, Mardinger O. Use of dental implants to improve unfavorable removable partial denture design. Compend Contin Educ Dent. 2005; 26:744-746, 748, 750 passim.

15. Mitrani R, Brudvik JS, Phillips KM. Posterior implants for distal extension removable prostheses: a retrospective study. Int J Periodontics Restorative Dent. 2003; 23:353-359.

16. Grossmann Y, Nissan J, Levin L. Clinical effectiveness of implant-supported removable partial dentures: a review of the literature and retrospective case evaluation. J Oral Maxillofac Surg. 2009; 67:1941-1946

17. Kaufmann R, Friedli M, Hug S, Mericske-Stern R. Removable dentures with implant support in strategic positions followed for up to 8 years. Int J Prosthodont. 2009; 22:233-241

18. Krennmair G, Krainhöfner M, Waldenberger O, Piehslinger E. Dental implants as strategic supplementary abutments for implant-tooth-supported telescopic crown-retained maxillary dentures: a retrospective follow-up study for up to 9 years. Int J Prosthodont. 2007; 20:617-622.

19. Mijiritsky E. Implants in conjunction with removable partial dentures: a literature review. Implant Dent 2007;16:146-154.

20. Payne AG, Tawse-Smith A, Wismeijer D, De Silva RK, Ma S. Multicentre prospective evaluation of implant-assisted mandibular removable partial dentures: surgical and prosthodontic outcomes. Clin Oral Implants Res. 2017;28:116-125.

21. Rinke S, Ziebolz D, Ratka-Krüger P, Frisch E. Clinical Outcome of Double Crown-Retained Mandibular Removable Dentures Supported by a Combination of Residual Teeth and Strategic Implants. J Prosthodont. 2015; 24:358-365.

22. Bernhart G, Koob A, Schmitter M, Gabbert O, Stober T, Rammelsberg P. Clinical success of implant-supported and tooth-implant-supported double crown-retained dentures. Clin Oral Investig. 2012;16:1031-1037.

23. Grossmann Y, Levin L, Sadan A. A retrospective case series of implants used to restore partially edentulous patients with implant-supported removable partial dentures: 31-month mean follow-up results. Quintessence Int. 2008;39:665-671.

24. Hug S, Mantokoudis D, Mericske-Stern R. Clinical evaluation of 3 overdenture concepts with tooth roots and implants: 2-year results. Int J Prosthodont. 2006;19:236-243.

25. Bae EB, Kim SJ, Choi JW, Jeon YC, Jeong CM, Yun MJ, Lee SH, Huh JB. A Clinical Retrospective Study of Distal Extension Removable Partial Denture with Implant Surveyed Bridge or Stud Type Attachment. Biomed Res Int. 2017;2017:7140870.

26. Cunha LD, Pellizzer EP, Verri FR, Pereira JA. Evaluation of the influence of location of osseointegrated implants associated with mandibular removable partial dentures. Implant Dent. 2008;17:278-287.

27. Verri FR, Pellizzer EP, Rocha EP, Pereira JA. Influence of length and diameter of implants associated with distal extension removable partial dentures. Implant Dent. 2007;16:270-280

28. de Freitas Santos CM, Pellizzer EP, Verri FR, de Moraes SL, Falcón-Antenucci RM. Influence of implant inclination associated with mandibular class I removable partial denture. J Craniofac Surg. 2011;22:663-668.

29. Pellizzer EP, Verri FR, Falcón-Antenucci RM, Goiato MC, Gennari Filho H. Evaluation of different retention systems on a distal extension removable partial denture associated with an osseointegrated implant. J Craniofac Surg. 2010;21:727-734.

30. Cunha LD, Pellizzer EP, Verri FR, Falcón-Antenucci RM, Goiato MC. Influence of ridge inclination and implant localization on the association of mandibular Kennedy class I removable partial denture. J Craniofac Surg. 2011;22:871-875.

31. Peroz I, Leuenberg A, Haustein I, Lange KP. Comparison between balanced occlusion and canine guidance in complete denture wearers--a clinical, randomized trial. Quintessence Int. 2003;34:607-612.

32. Oh YK, Bae EB, Huh JB. Retrospective clinical evaluation of implant-assisted removable partial dentures combined with implant surveyed prostheses. J Prosthet Dent. 2020 Aug 10;S0022-3913(20)30297-3. Online ahead of print.

33. Kang SH, Kim SK, Heo SJ, Koak JY. Survival rate and clinical evaluation of the implants in implant assisted removable partial dentures: surveyed crown and overdenture. J Adv Prosthodont. 2020;12:239-249.

# What are the roles of teeth and implants in an RPD?

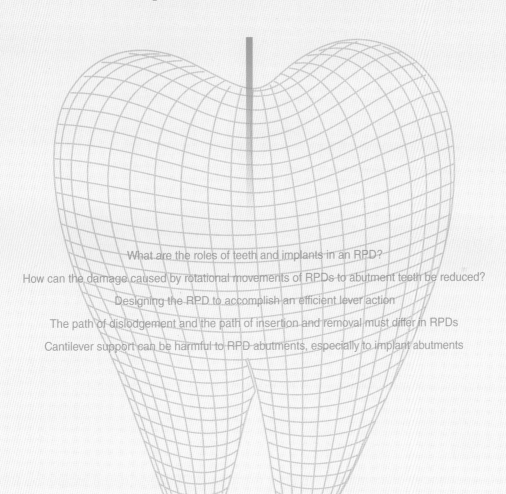

# What are the roles of teeth and implants in an RPD?

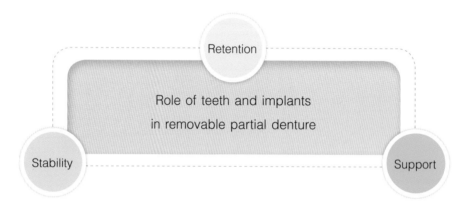

**Figure 1 :** Role of teeth and implants in removable partial denture or overdenture.

The role of teeth and implants in dentures is to provide retention, support, and stability.

### Question

**A patient experiences discomfort in his/her mandibular bilateral distal extension RPD**

*Patient : Doctor, my lower denture feels unstable whenever I chew, and it makes my rear gums hurt.*

*Doctor : Oh dear, your denture has bad retention. We will have to make you a new one.*

### Answer

A lack of support and stability makes the RPD move downward whenever the patient bites and this is why the distally extended edentulous site may hurt. It is not due to a lack of retention.

Retention prevents the dentures from being lifted away from the residual ridges. Support prevents dentures from being pressed down towards the residual ridges. Both retention and support resist the vertical movements of dentures. In contrast, stability is responsible for resisting the non-vertical movements of RPDs.

The most important element in designing RPDs is providing support. When learning how to design RPDs for the first time, the procedure for fabricating tooth-supported and tooth- and tissue-supported RPDs are taught separately because establishment of support differs in the two types. The next important element that needs to be considered is stability. If a patient complains of denture movement during mastication, it is because the RPD lacks support and stability. On the other hand, if the RPD lacks retention, the patient would complain that the denture falls out too easily.

> **Keypoint**
>
> It is incorrect to adjust clasps to fix an unstable, mobile RPD. Clasps are responsible for the retention of dentures, and it is important to minimize the forces induced by the clasps.

**Question**

**In the following figure, which components of the RPD metal framework provide support, retention, and stability?**

**Answer**

Figure 2 illustrates the different components of the RPD metal framework and their roles in providing support, retention and stability.

Support : No.1 (blue) - Cingulum and occlusal rests

Retention : No.2 (orange) - Retentive clasp arms

Stability : No.3 (yellow) - Minor connectors (proximal plates, located at the mesial or distal end of the abutment tooth, are particularly important), and the reciprocal arm at palatal area of the second molar

No.4 (green) - Major connector (in the maxilla, a major connector covering the palate can provide additional support to the RPD)

Others : No.5 (grey) - Minor connectors connected to the denture base.

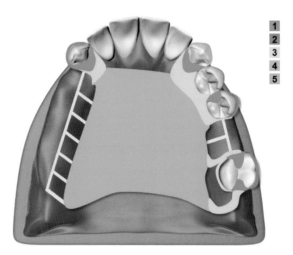

**Figure 2.** Components of the RPD metal framework and their main roles. 1: support, 2: retention, 3-5: stability

---

**Keypoint**

When there are a sufficient number of intact teeth or implants, it is possible to assign the support, retention, and stability elements to those teeth or implants. However, when the number of teeth or implants decreases, all three elements, support, retention, and stability, need to be assigned to the RPD itself. Thus, if there are a sufficient number of teeth or implants, the RPD design itself can provide support, retention, and stability. If this is not the case, additional support and stability can be provided by proper impression taking. If stability is still insufficient, additional stability can be provided through occlusion, such as bilateral balanced occlusion.

---

The important thing to keep in mind is, when only a few teeth or implants are left to provide support, retention, and stability to the RPD, they are likely to have poor prognoses.

**Question**

## What are the roles of teeth or implants in the following treatment (Figure 3)?

**Answer**

A 53-year old female patient presented with discomfort from her existing mandibular bilateral distal extension RPD. She was pursuing aesthetic prostheses at a minimal cost without a bone graft. Her mandibular teeth had first degree mobility. She was treated with a cross arch splint after periodontal treatment of the remaining teeth. Implants were placed on both first premolars with attachments, rest seats were placed on

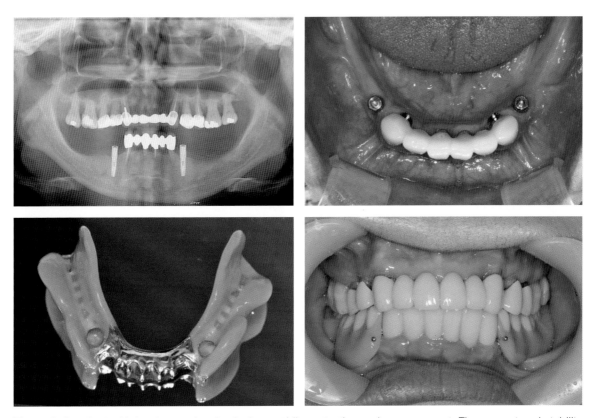

**Figure 3.** A patient with locators on two implants, providing retention and some support. The support and stability are provided by the remaining teeth and are maximized with the denture base.

the lingual surface of the remaining mandibular canines, and a bilateral distal extension RPD was fabricated.

The patient had poor periodontal health, resulting in first degree mobility of mandibular incisors. Implants were placed on both first premolar areas with locator attachments taking into account the condition of the remaining teeth as well as aesthetics. In this case, the locator attachments mainly provide retention, and thus clasps were not required. Because the remaining teeth were periodontically unhealthy, a cross arch splint was placed. In addition, rest seats were formed on both canines to form a lingual plate. This was done to provide vertical support and stability to the remaining teeth. The rests provided support, and distal proximal plates on abutment teeth provided stability. By not using clasps on the teeth, harmful forces such as a lateral force can be prevented. In order to decrease the harmful stress exerted on the implants, the locators were designed to function as retentive and supportive elements. Unfortunately, however, the remaining teeth were too weak to provide sufficient stability in this case. Therefore, the occlusion and impression taking method provided additional stability. In other words, achieving a bilateral balanced occlusion and extending the denture base sufficiently would have provided additional stability

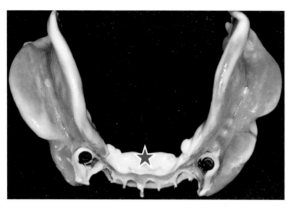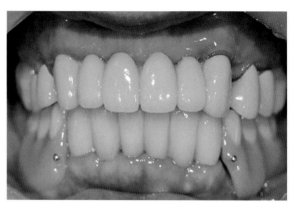

**Figure 4.** Stability and support are obtained from a sufficiently extended, well-fitting denture.

★ fit checker

to protect the weak remaining teeth (Figure 4). How stability is provided by the occlusion and denture base will be covered in later chapters.

---

**Keypoint**

**In the case of Figure 3, support, retention, and stability are provided by the following areas:**

**Support** – rest seats on teeth, locators, buccal shelf area from a sufficiently extended denture base

**Retention** – two locators

**Stability** – distal proximal plate on the remaining abutment teeth, sufficiently extended lingual denture base, bilateral balanced occlusion, well-fitting denture base

---

# REFERENCES

1.  Berg T, Caputo AA. Anterior rests for maxillary removable partial dentures. The Journal of prosthetic dentistry. 1978;39:139-146.

2.  Henderson D. Major connectors for removable partial dentures: design and function. The Journal of prosthetic dentistry 1973;30:532-548.

3.  Fisher RL, Jaslow C. The efficiency of an indirect retainer. The Journal of prosthetic dentistry. 1975;34:24-30.

4.  Fisher RL. Factors that influence the base stability of mandibular distal-extension removable partial dentures: A longitudinal study. The Journal of prosthetic dentistry. 1983;50:167-171.

5.  Frank RP. Direct retainers for distal-extension removable partial dentures. The Journal of prosthetic dentistry. 1986;56:562-567.

6.  Grossmann Y, Nissan J, Levin L. Clinical effectiveness of implant-supported removable partial dentures-a review of the literature and retrospective case evaluation. Journal of Oral and Maxillofacial Surgery. 2009;67:1941-1946.

7.  Igarashi Y, Ogata A, Kuroiwa A, Wang CH. Stress distribution and abutment tooth mobility of distal-extension removable partial dentures with different retainers: an in vivo study. Journal of oral rehabilitation. 1999;26:111-116.

8.  Lytle RB. Soft tissue displacement beneath removable partial and complete dentures. The Journal of Prosthetic Dentistry. 1962;12:34-43.

9.  Ohkubo C, Kobayashi M, Suzuki Y, Hosoi T. Effect of implant support on distal-extension removable partial dentures: in vivo assessment. International Journal of Oral & Maxillofacial Implants. 2008:23:1095-1101.

10. Suenaga H, Kubo K, Hosokawa R, Kuriyagawa T, Sasaki K. Effects of Occlusal Rest Design on Pressure Distribution Beneath the Denture Base of a Distal Extension Removable Partial Denture-An In Vivo Study. International Journal of Prosthodontics. 2014;27:469-471.

*Chapter 2-2.*

# How can the damage caused by rotational movements of RPDs to abutment teeth be reduced?

If a dentist is not aware of the different types of RPD movements, he or she may blindly hand over the fabrication process to a dental technician, whose job is to design a denture, without being aware of the conditions of the patient.

Before discussing the various types of RPD movements, the RPD classification must be understood. Even with the same case, the RPD movements can be entirely different depending on how the RPD is classified. Consequently, the RPD can be designed to prevent such movements.

### Question

**What is the Kennedy classification in Figure 1?**

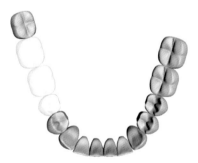

**Figure 1.** The lower right third molar remains while the lower right second premolar as well as the first and second molars on the same side are missing.

Answer

In this case, there is no single correct answer. If the lower right third molar is included in the RPD, that is, if a clasp assembly is designed on it, the denture would be classified as Kennedy Class III. However, if the edentulous area is extensive, and the lower right third molar abutment tooth is in poor condition (if the abutment tooth has a slight mobility), the denture should be designed to provide support from the edentulous area. Because tooth-supported RPDs and tooth- and tissue-supported RPDs undergo different movements, the designs must also differ.

> **Keypoint**
>
> When classifying patients, dentists should consider two types of classification systems.
> : Kennedy and Beckett (similar to the system suggested by Bailyn) classifications. The Kennedy classification is determined by the edentulous state, and the Beckett classification is determined by the degree of support.

## (1) Kennedy Classification

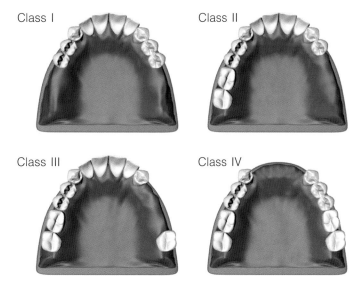

Class I     Class II

Class III     Class IV

**Figure 2.** The Kennedy classification system.

Kennedy Class I: Bilateral free-end saddles (Bilateral distal extension RPD).

Kennedy Class II: Unilateral free-end saddle (Unilateral distal extension RPD).

Kennedy Class III: Unilateral bounded saddle; support is given to the teeth adjacent to the edentulous area.

Kennedy Class IV: Anterior bounded saddle; this classification is given only when left and right anterior teeth are missing.

The posterior-most edentulous area determines the type of Kennedy classification. Any other edentulous areas are used to determine the modification.

### Question

**What is the Kennedy Classification of the figure below?**

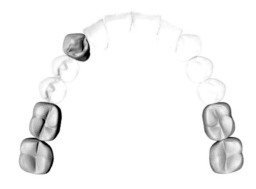

**Figure 3.** Kennedy class III modification I

### Answer

The figure above displays a Kennedy Class III modification 1. Although it may appear like a Kennedy Class IV denture due to many missing anterior teeth, it is a Kennedy Class III because the upper right first and second premolars are the most posterior region of the edentulous area. A Kennedy Class III is generally known as a tooth-supported RPD. However, can the figure above truly represent a tooth-supported RPD? Due to the extensive anterior edentulous area, should it not have tissue support?

As we can see from this case, the Kennedy classification alone cannot determine the design of the RPD. Therefore, along with the Kennedy classification, the degree of tissue support should also be considered.

### (2) Beckett Classification based on the support of dentures

Class I: Tooth-supported

Class II: Tissue-supported

Class III: Tooth- and tissue-supported

> **Keypoint**
>
> The Kennedy Classification system alone cannot determine the appropriate design for an RPD. The course of treatment for patients should be determined considering all the other factors.

**Two different RPD designs are depicted below.**

**What is the difference? Why are they designed in such a manner?**

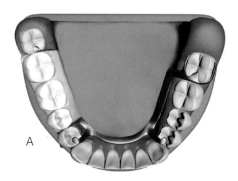 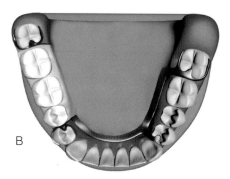

A                                                   B

**Figure 4.** Understanding the design of a Kennedy Class II and III.

**Answer**

### Figure 4A

This displays a Kennedy Class III RPD, but it is expected to be converted to a Kennedy Class II, a tooth- and tissue-supported RPD, in the future. Even if there are teeth with slight mobility resulting from poor periodontal conditions, extraction may not be possible immediately. As such, the teeth are less resistant to lateral forces but can withstand some degree of vertical force. Therefore, when the prognosis of the lower right third molar is poor and the transition to a Kennedy Class II is expected in a relatively short time period, the initial design can simply be a Kennedy Class II denture. A mesial rest can be placed on the lower right third molar (while a proximal plate and a clasp may be omitted) to minimize the lateral or rotational force on the abutment tooth, and to provide vertical support for the denture. Placing an RPI (Rest-Proximal plate-I bar) clasp on the lower right first premolar and a rest on the lower left first premolar as an indirect retainer, would accommodate the functional movement of the denture. The roles of clasps and indirect retainers will be discussed later in more detail.

### Figure 4B

If the lower right third molar is in a very good condition with the proper undercut for a clasp, design a Kennedy Class III, a tooth-supported RPD. There is no need for the RPI or RPA (Rest-Proximal plate-Akers) clasp, which accommodate functional movement in tooth- and tissue-supported RPDs. A distal rest and a circumferential clasp should be placed on the lower right first premolar. Unlike in Figure 4A, the rest on the lower left first premolar is not an indirect retainer but provides support by distributing the vertical stress of the RPD. Additional stability is obtained by the minor connectors.

**What are the possible movements in a tooth- and tissue-supported RPD? How is it different from a tooth-supported RPD?**

In addition to support and retention, the teeth and implants also provide stability. Usually, an RPD is subjected to three types of rotational movements as shown in Figure 5. The first is a rotational movement about the fulcrum line passing through the most posterior abutment teeth, when the denture base moves vertically towards or away from the supporting residual ridge. The second is a rotational movement about the longitudinal axis formed by the crest of the residual ridge. The third is a rotational movement about the vertical axis located on the virtual center of the arch.

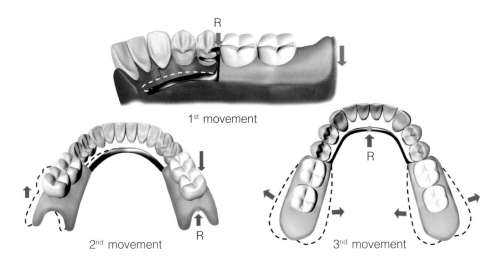

1st movement

2nd movement

3nd movement

**Figure 5.** Three types of rotational movements that disturb the stability of the denture. The first movement usually occurs due to weak vertical support from the edentulous residual ridge and the absence of an indirect retainer in the anterior of the fulcrum line.

In a tooth (or an implant)-supported RPD, the tooth or implant prevents all three movements, and the RPD design becomes very simplistic. However, if the tooth or implant cannot prevent these rotations, a rotational axis is formed to generate rotational movements. In other words, unintended rotational movements may occur in a tooth- and tissue-supported RPD, exerting harmful stress on abutment teeth or implants.

As shown in Figures 6A and B, stability is not a major concern for RPDs held by four teeth or implants, because the axes of rotation are not formed by the teeth or implants. However, a denture held by only two implants has a definite axis of rotation and rotates around it. If two implant attachments are used, as

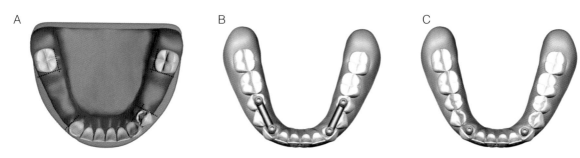

**Figure 6.** Stability is obtained according to the number of teeth and implants. A: a tooth-supported RPD, B: 4-implants overdenture, C: 2-implants overdenture

shown in Figure 6C, a functional impression should be taken on the posterior edentulous area in order to prevent vertical denture movement towards the residual ridge. If necessary, appropriate occlusion (e.g. bilateral balanced occlusion) should be created to minimize the rotational movements around the implants that may occur during mastication, and to prolong the life span of the attachments.

> **Keypoint**
>
> An overdenture using two implants has to take into account more factors compared to a complete denture. A definite rotational movement occurs around the implants, and if the denture itself does not have sufficient support and stability, excessive stress is exerted on the implants.

**Question**

**What is the difference in overdenture movements when implants are placed at different locations or have different attachments?**

**Answer**

In Figure 7, the difference between A and B is the distance between the two anterior and two posterior implants. The distance is greater in B than A. In other words, the anterior to posterior spread (A-P spread) differs. The longer the A-P spread of the overdenture, the more likely it will become an implant-supported RPD, which blocks tissue-ward movement of the distal extension area. The smaller the A-P spread, the more likely it will become an implant-retentive RPD, which allows tissue-ward movement of the distal extension area. Since both A and B used only one clip at the anterior bar, the first movement, as displayed in Figure 7, may occur. Figure 7B represents more posterior support (as compared with Figure 7A), suggesting less occurrence of the first movement under the precondition that the posterior implant

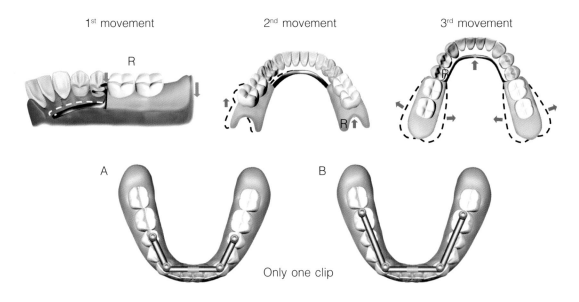

1st movement     2nd movement     3rd movement

A     B

Only one clip

**Figure 7.** The different movement of an overdenture retained by a bar and a clip according to the implant location.

is in contact with the denture base. Furthermore, the second and third movements will also be reduced.

As shown in Figure 8, four implants with bars are located in the same position for both A and B. However, if the number of clips change, the movement of the overdenture will also differ. In B, where the overdenture has three clips, all three movements will therefore be significantly reduced.

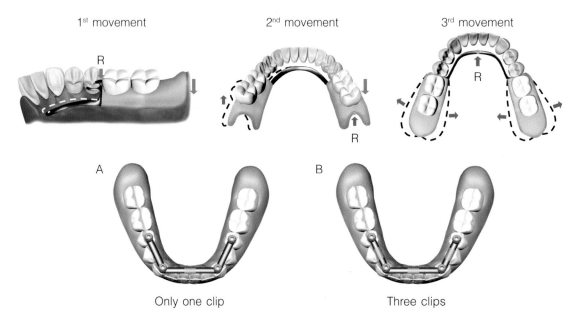

1st movement     2nd movement     3rd movement

A     B

Only one clip     Three clips

**Figure 8.** The various movements of overdentures depending on the number of clips used.

As learned from Figures 7 and 8, even with the same number of implants, overdenture movement can vary depending on the location of the implants and the number and type of attachments. In addition, reduced denture movement indicates that most of the rotational forces have been transferred to the implants. This is similar to a tooth-supported RPD. Taken together then, how does Figure 8B compare with Figure 8A? As seen in Figure 8B, all the rotational forces are concentrated on the implants, and there may be no tissue support in the posterior edentulous area, creating a cantilever anchored by the anterior implants and clips. However, as seen in Figure 8A, where tissue-ward movements of the distal extension base are allowed, the forces are distributed to the implants and the residual ridges.

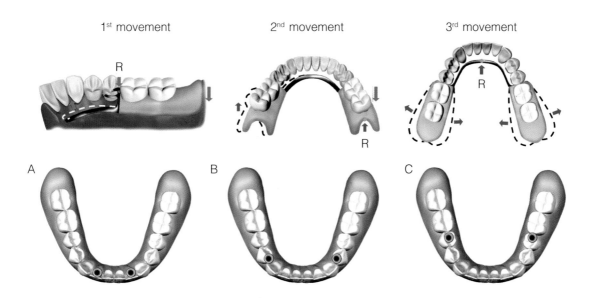

**Figure 9.** The three different movements in two-implant-overdentures with locator attachments according to their implant locations.

If we assume that two implants are located in different locations as shown in Figures 9A, B, and C, how are their movements differentiated? Movements may vary depending on the type of attachment, but let's suppose we use locators in this case. Locators provide support and retention, and may also have resistance against lateral forces. Assuming the dentures are identical, the first movement may increase in degree from A to C and the second and third movements may decrease in degree from A to C (see Chapter 4.5).

## What is the meaning of vertical retention and support on implants and teeth?

In general, the clasp assembly is composed of a rest, a minor connector, a retention arm, and a reciprocal arm. These components are similar to the parts of a screw as shown in Figure 10.

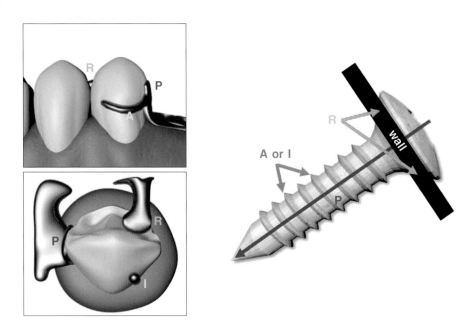

**Figure 10.** Similarity between a clasp assembly and a screw.

In Figure 10, A and I represent retention of the clasp. The proximal plate of the RPD serves as the path of insertion. The head of the screw can be regarded as a rest that provides support while it is contacting the wall. The principles of removable prostheses are similar to that of fixing frames to the ceiling.

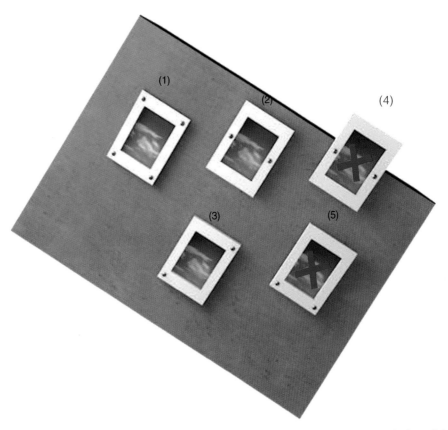

**Figure 11.** The principle of hanging frames on the ceiling using screws helps to explain the design of the RPD.

As shown in Figure 11, we are going to hang five frames on the ceiling. Frame (1) is fixed with four screws, one at each corner, fixing it to the ceiling very firmly. Let's say we are given only two screws to hang the frames, as shown in (2) and (3). Compared to frame (1), they seem relatively unstable, but they are still well-fixated. In frame (5) on the other hand, two screws are fixed on the corners of one side. Like frames (2) and (3), two screws are used, but frame (5) is more unstable than frames (2) and (3). If you pull the upper side of frame (5), it could easily fall from the ceiling. Frame (4), as in frame (2), is fixed in the middle with two screws, with the upper half protruding beyond the ceiling edge, pressing on the upper side would likely detach the frame from the ceiling. The wall (supporting factor) under the frame located anterior to the axis of rotation along the screws serves as an indirect retainer. In other words, frames (2) and (3) are supported by the wall anterior to the axis of rotation along the screws. As a result, when the frame rotates and tries to fall off, the screw tries to pull out vertically so it can resist the pulling force more efficiently. In frames (4) and (5), there is no wall to support the frames, so when they rotate around the axis of rotation, the screws are twisted and the frames easily fall.

> **Keypoint**
>
> The role of an indirect retainer is to help the direct retainer be removed as vertically as possible using the rigid support located anterior to the direct retainer.

This principle can be applied directly to RPDs. Figure 12 compares Kennedy Class II and III RPDs with frames.

The upper left image in Figure 12 shows a tooth (or an implant)-supported RPD. The teeth are fully supportive and have four stable clasp assemblies. It acts in the same way as a frame fixed by four screws. Solid support is obtained from the teeth, we can assume that the wall under the frame is a very hard concrete wall. Thus, in this case, there is no need to consider other designs. It is not necessary to make an indirect retainer in the front since there is no need to worry about potential rotation. Keeping the occlusion coherent with the remaining teeth, simply take an impression of the anatomical form. The image on the bottom right in Figure 12 shows a frame fixed with three screws. It seems quite stable, despite having only three screws. Eventually, as shown in the upper right image in Figure 12, the upper left first

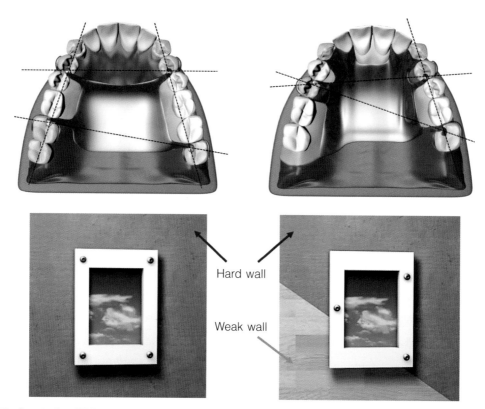

**Figure 12.** Comparing RPD designs and frames. Hard wall is a solid support like rest of tooth, weak wall is a resilient support like soft tissue of edentulous area.

premolar becomes an indirect retainer; it is possible to make a stable RPD without the need to consider an additional indirect retainer. However, the edentulous area on the upper right posterior part can be thought of as a weak wall (plywood). The weak wall can be slightly compressed, so there is a possibility that the clasp pulls on the upper left first premolar every time the patient chews on the upper right side. If this is the case, you can take a functional impression of the edentulous area on the upper right side to provide enough support, replace the upper left first premolar clasp with a wrought wire or omit a clasp.

As shown in Figure 13, if there is a weak wall in the posterior region, the frame rotates due to a vertical external force. As a result of this repetitive rotational movement, the screws on the opposite side of the axis of rotation is repeatedly pulled out and loosened, and eventually, the screw in the middle will be removed. Similar to screws, teeth, and implants are also weak against a twisting torque. Thus, if a denture is easily removed, or a twisting torque is transmitted directly to an abutment tooth or implant, it is more vulnerable to damage. It is important to minimize this rotational movement in order to ensure a long-term prognosis of the implants in an IARPD.

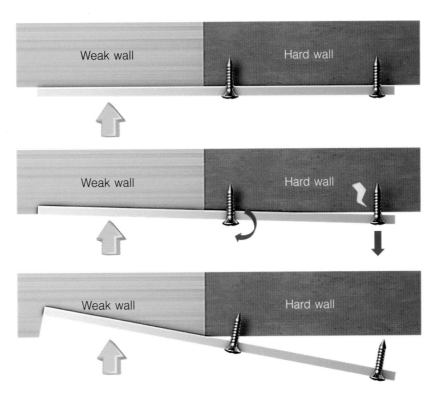

**Figure 13.** Rotational movement of the frame when there is a weak wall.

Unlike Figure 14A, Figure 14C shows how to design an indirect retainer using three screws in unilaterally edentulous cases (indicated by the red arrow). In this case, it is not necessary to design a clasp on the upper left first premolar. Instead, only a minimal amount of retention is needed to prevent the denture from being displaced vertically. If the clasp is misplaced and there is less support in edentulous area, a pulling force on the abutment tooth may occur every time the patient chews. The rest on the upper left first premolar becomes a rigid wall, which serves as an indirect retainer and helps the direct retainers of the upper right first premolar and upper left second molar to be dislodge vertically. This concept is easier to understand if you think about the rotation with or without the rest on the upper left first premolar.

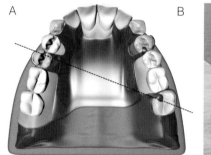 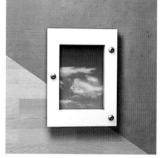 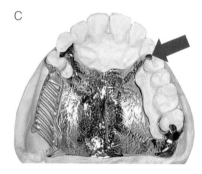

**Figure 14.** A, B, and C (from left to right). In order to insert three screws, an indirect retainer is designed on the upper left first premolar in the unilateral distal extension case.

Figure 15 shows RPD designs depending on the position of direct retainers when there are only two of them. Since the posterior edentulous area becomes a weak wall, it is better to minimize movement by taking a functional impression, and if possible, placing the direct retainers in the center of the frame. Also, it would be best to make an indirect retainer on the teeth anterior to the most posterior axis of rotation. Keep in mind that designing a rest on a tooth is equivalent to creating a rigid wall under the frame, and it is this wall that makes the denture displace vertically.

> **Keypoint**
>
> Indirect retainers provide vertical support as well as help direct retainers to dislodge vertically.

The design of indirect retainers can limit the movements of RPD in one direction. Take, for example, Figure 15A. If there is no indirect retainer, a seesaw movement occurs in the anterior-posterior direction

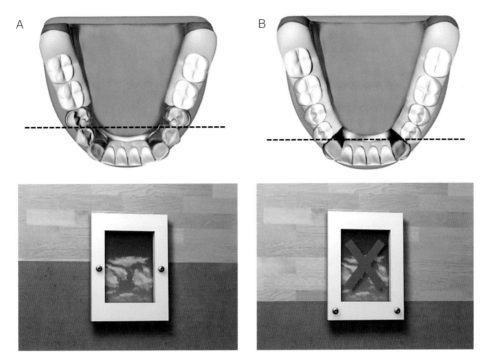

**Figure 15.** Stability of frames according to the position of two screws. As shown in A, the cingulum rests on both canines serve as indirect retainers (a rigid wall under the frame) that helps the clasps on both second premolars to be displaced vertically.

around the posterior-most abutment teeth. However, if there is an indirect retainer, an upward movement occurs in the posterior RPD. In other words, it becomes easy to control such movements. Then the only thing to consider is how to deal with the potentially harmful forces caused by the posterior downward movement.

# REFERENCES

1. Avant WE. Fulcrum and retention lines in planning removable partial dentures. J Prosthet Dent. 1971;25:162-166.

2. Avant WE. Indirect retention in partial denture design. 1966. J Prosthet Dent. 2003;90:1-5.

3. Beckett LS. Practical and effective designs for removable partial prostheses. Australian dental journal. 1965;10:239-248.

4. Bural C, Buzbas B, Ozatik S, Bayraktar G, Emes Y. Distal extension mandibular removable partial denture with implant support. European Journal of Dentistry. 2016;10:566-570.

5. Cecconi BT, Asgar K, Dootz E. The effect of partial denture clasp design on abutment tooth movement. J Prosthet Dent. 197;25:44-56.

6. Cecconi BT, Asgar K, Dootz E. clasp assembly modifications and their effect on abutment tooth movement. J Prosthet Dent. 1972;27:160-167.

7. Eliason CM. RPA clasp design for distal-extension removable partial dentures. J Prosthet Dent. 1983;49:25-27.

8. Fisher RL, Jaslow C. The efficiency of an indirect retainer. The Journal of prosthetic dentistry. 1975;34:24-30.

9. Frank RP, Nicholls JI. An investigation of the effectiveness of indirect retainers. The Journal of prosthetic dentistry. 1977;38:494-506.

10. Grossmann Y, Nissan J, Levin L. Clinical effectiveness of implant-supported removable partial dentures—a review of the literature and retrospective case evaluation. Journal of Oral and Maxillofacial Surgery. 2009;67:1941-1946.

11. Jensen C, Meijer HJA, Raghoebar GM, Kerdijk W, Cune MS. Implant-supported removable partial dentures in the mandible: A 3-16 year retrospective study J Prosthodont Res. 2017;61:98-105.

12. Krol AJ. clasp design for extension-base removable partial dentures. J Prosthet Dent. 1973;29:408-415.

13. Kuzmanovic DV, Payne AG, Purton DG. Distal implants to modify the Kennedy classification of a removable partial denture: a clinical report. The Journal of prosthetic dentistry. 2004;92:8-11.

14. Matsudate Y1, Yoda N2, Nanba M1, Ogawa T1, Sasaki K Load distribution on abutment tooth, implant and residual ridge with distal-extension implant-supported removable partial denture. J Prosthodont Res. 2016;60:282-288.

15. McDowell GC, Fisher RL. Force transmission by indirect retainers when a unilateral dislodging force is applied. The Journal of prosthetic dentistry. 1982;47:360-365.

16. McGarry TJ, Nimmo A, Skiba JF, Ahlstrom RH, Smith CR, Koumjian JH, Arbree NS. Classification system for partial edentulism. Journal of Prosthodontics. 2002;11:181-193.

17. Miller EL. Systems for classifying partially dentulous arches. J Prosthet Dent. 1970;24:25-40.

18. Mitrani R, Brudvik JS, Phillips KM. Posterior implants for distal extension removable prostheses: a retrospective study. International Journal of Periodontics & Restorative Dentistry. 2003;23:352-359.

19. Sato M, Suzuki Y, Kurihara D, Shimpo H, Ohkubo C. Effect of implant support on mandibular distal extension

removable partial dentures: relationship between denture supporting area and stress distribution. Journal of prosthodontic research. 2013;57:109-112.

20. William E. Factors that influence retention of removable partial dentures. J Prosthet Dent. 1971;25: 265-270.

Chapter 2-3.

# Designing the RPD to accomplish an efficient lever action

Tooth- and tissue-supported RPDs are distinct from other types of prostheses such as tooth-supported RPDs, fixed partial dentures, and complete dentures in that a definite fulcrum line can be identified. Depending on the location of the fulcrum line, various types of denture movements can be generated. Particularly, when both teeth and implants are used as abutments of RPDs, it is crucial to understand how to control all the physical forces applied to the abutments and how to prevent any adverse rotational forces from being applied to the implants by the RPDs.

### Question

**How are tooth-supported RPDs and tooth- and tissue-supported RPDs different in terms of their support and stress distribution?**

### Answer

The term 'tooth-supported' in this book implies support from both implants and teeth.

A well-fabricated fixed partial denture on teeth or implants is structurally capable of withstanding axial and non-axial forces. Edentulous parts are supported by abutment teeth at each end so that the majority of the occlusal force is transferred vertically to the abutment teeth, thus minimizing any harmful rotational forces.

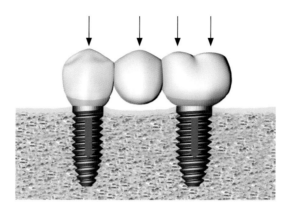

**Figure 1.** Distribution of forces in tooth (implant)-supported fixed partial dentures.

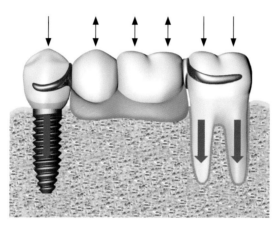

**Figure 2.** Distribution of forces in tooth-supported RPDs involving both teeth and implant abutments.

Just as in fixed partial dentures, tooth-supported (Kennedy Class III) RPDs receive support solely from the abutment teeth at each end. In RPDs, occlusal forces are transferred vertically along the long axis of the abutment teeth as depicted in Figure 2. This can be addressed by properly designed rest seats and proximal plates. However, as it is a removable prosthesis, there is always the potential that rotational forces are exerted on the abutment teeth.

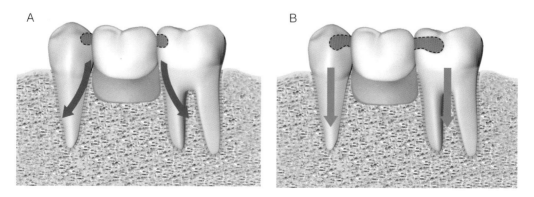

**Figure 3.** Distribution of forces in different shapes of rest seats.

As depicted in Figure 3A, a short rest is placed on the tooth margin, exerting an unwanted force that is not parallel to the long axis of the abutment teeth. Therefore, an occlusal rest must be appropriately designed in order to transfer the load in the axial direction and prevent injury to the periodontal ligament of the teeth or impairment to the osseointegration of implant fixtures. As depicted in Figure 3B, a rest must be extended further into the occlusal surface at an acute angle to the minor connector (proximal plate) in order to convert the exerted force to a vertical direction.

Imagine a Kennedy Class I RPD with an implant surveyed crown, as depicted in Figure 4; non-axial forces are applied to the abutment whenever an occlusal force is exerted. The distal extension RPD base shows a larger range of displacement than the implant-supported fixed dental prostheses. While natural

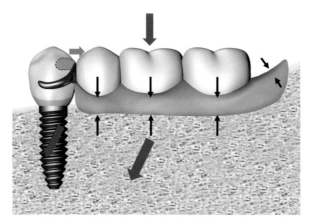

**Figure 4.** Distribution of forces in a Kennedy Class I RPD with an implant surveyed crown.

teeth can rely on protection from the periodontal ligament, implants are more vulnerable to rotational forces that can bring about further complications. The denture base rotates around the rest that is adjacent to the edentulous area, and this rotational force is consistently exerted distally on the abutment.

In cases in which the anterior teeth are missing (Figure 5), the anterior denture base supported by the underlying soft tissue shows a larger displacement than the abutment teeth supported by the periodontal ligament. If the abutment is an implant, the prognosis of the implant would be questionable. If it is a natural tooth, the abutment tooth may be tilted towards the mesial side to widen the interdental space and may also result in tooth mobility.

These problems occur more often to implants than teeth since the acceptable range of movement of implant prostheses is limited than as compared to of teeth.

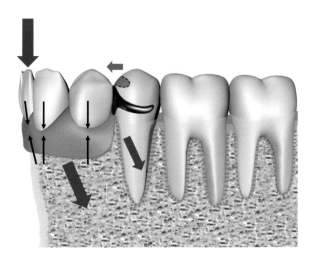

Figure 5. Distribution of forces in a Kennedy Class IV RPD..

> **Keypoint**
>
> In an IARPD, it is important to avoid exerting adverse forces on implants by the lever actions of the RPD. The lever actions that remain unresolved even after designing the metal framework can be dealt with by taking a functional impression and creating a bilateral balanced occlusion, which can adjunctively minimize denture movements.

**Question**

## Why is it important to understand the principles of a lever when designing RPDs?

**Answer**

The ultimate goal of designing RPDs is to prevent any harmful Class I lever actions and to accommodate efficient lever actions during mastication so that adverse forces on the abutments are minimized. Typically, Class I levers in distal extension RPDs act to exert harmful rotational forces on the abutments. When Class I lever is unavoidable, adjusting the point of load, fulcrum, and effort (or force), is required to minimize the force transferred to the abutment. To do so, the lever actions must be understood thoroughly.

RPDs transfer the occlusal load to the intraoral tissues following two basic mechanical principles. As seen in Figure 6, a vertical force, E, is exerted on the yellow object on the ramp, and the object slides down the ramp as a consequence. The levers beneath the ramp diagram show that work is done by rotating about the fulcrum (F) upon the exertion of a vertical downward force (E), moving (L) on the other end upwards. Carefully observe the two figures and notice how the force applied in one direction can be transferred to unintended areas. Clinically, we must prevent the transfer of these harmful forces exerted on abutments by limiting denture movements.

## (1) Class I lever

A class I lever has the fulcrum placed between the effort and the load.

This lever is applied when you want to lift a heavy object. The further the effort from the fulcrum, the

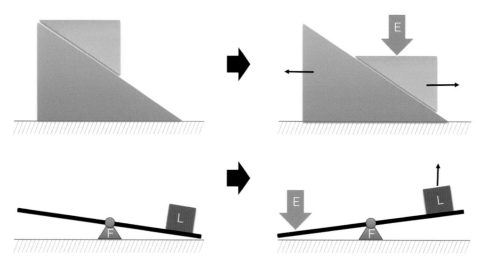

**Figure 6.** A force applied in one direction can be unintentionally transferred to other unwanted directions.

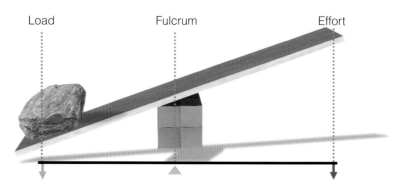

**Figure 7.** A seesaw is analogous to a Class I lever action.

better the efficiency of the lever. When a Class I action lever is unavoidable in an RPD, the distance from the fulcrum to the load can be adjusted to minimize the adverse rotational force exerted on the abutment.

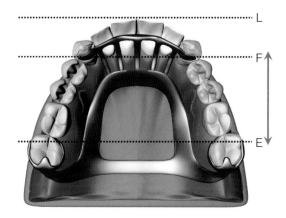

**Figure 8.** Understanding Class I levers in a Kennedy Class IV RPD.

Figure 8 shows an RPD designed to maximize the efficiency of Class I levers. The fulcrum (F) is established upon the rests at either end of the anterior edentulous area. Therefore, as the patient tries to take a bite of an apple, for example, the load (L) is applied on the anterior artificial teeth. The edentulous area on the maxillary anterior part will be pressed by the denture base, which rotates about the fulcrum line. At this point, the clasps on the most posterior teeth work as the effort (E) to hold back this rotation. Clasps further away from the fulcrum can accommodate a Class I lever that is maximized in efficiency to withstand the load transferred to the teeth. If the posterior-most clasp (E) is moved anteriorly as shown

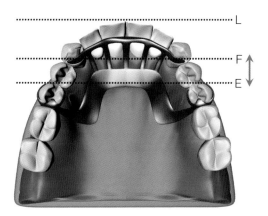

**Figure 9.** Understanding Class I levers in a Kennedy Class IV RPD. When the posterior-most clasps (E) are moved anteriorly, stronger retention is required on the anterior artificial teeth to withstand the same load.

in Figure 9, stronger retention would be required on the posterior clasp to withstand the same load on the anterior artificial teeth.

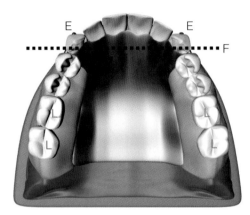

**Figure 10.** The adverse consequences of Class I levers on a Kennedy Class I RPD. Occlusal force (L) is applied to the posterior teeth leading to the rotational movement of the distal extension along the fulcrum line (F) and the pulling force of the clasp anterior to the fulcrum line. The rotational displacement of the distal extension RPD base increases with posterior alveolar resorption, leading to harmful lateral forces being exerted on the abutment teeth during mastication.

At first glance, it may appear that the design shown in Figure 8 is more favorable due to its ability to efficiently prevent rotational movements about the fulcrum with minimal effort from the posterior clasp, in turn exerting a minimal external force on the abutment. The retention (E) provided by the posterior abutment teeth, represented in Figures 8 and 9, is also called 'cantilevered support' (see Chapter 2.5). Class I levers in an RPD typically generate adverse rotational denture movements. For instance, in the Kennedy Class I RPD represented in Figure 10, the fulcrum line (F) lies on the posterior-most rests on the upper left and right canines, and the force (L) is loaded on the posterior teeth during mastication. The distal extension RPD is supported by the underlying soft tissue. Unfortunately, it is not firm enough to prevent the denture base from submerging, which in turn generates a rotational Class I lever action to transfer the occlusal force (L) to the clasps on the other side of the fulcrum. The force (E) applied on the clasps will exert consistent torsional stress on the abutment teeth, which is particularly harmful to the implant of IARPD.

### (2) Class II lever

A class II lever has the load placed between the fulcrum and the effort.

This type of lever is favorable, the load is always located closer to the fulcrum than the effort, thus there

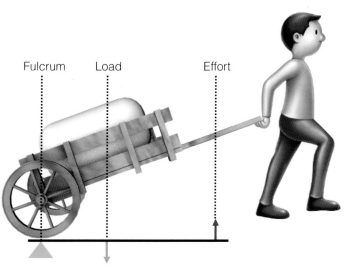

**Figure 11.** Understanding Class II levers. The load is always closer to the fulcrum than the effort.

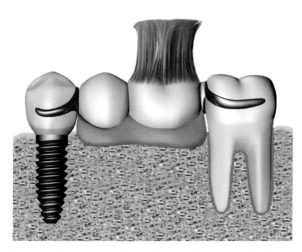

**Figure 12.** An example of how a Class II lever is activated. Note that this figure can be interpreted as either a Class II or Class III lever. In this book, a lever is determined from the perspective of the clasp, where the clasp is thought to 'make the effort'. In the figure above, the clasp acts as the 'effort' and the dislodging force of the chewing gum acts as the 'load', making it a Class II lever. However, if it is said that the chewing gum acts as the 'effort' and the dislodging force of the Clasp acts as the 'load', it would be a class III lever.

is no loss. In other words, a load of 100 will always be counteracted by an effort that is less than 100.

Imagine there is a piece of chewing gum stuck to the artificial molar tooth as shown in Figure 12. The hinge point lies on the rest of the first premolar implant abutment. Assume that the chewing gum is creating a dislodging force during the opening of the mouth to act as the load, and the clasp on the second molar works in the opposite direction to prevent the denture from dislodging. Class II levers have the load located between the fulcrum and the effort, making it possible to manage bigger loads with less effort from the retentive clasp.

### (3) Class III lever

Class III levers have the effort located between the load and the fulcrum. It is analogous to a castle drawbridge (Figures 13 and 14). Class III levers need a larger effort to counteract the load. As such, class III levers can be well utilized in tooth- and tissue-supported distal extension RPDs.

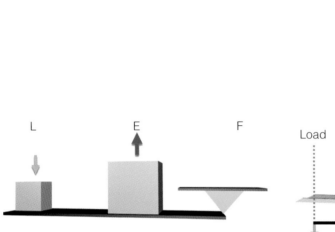

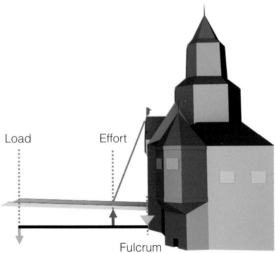

**Figure 13.** Understanding Class III levers. The effort is placed between the load and the fulcrum.

**Figure 14.** A Class III lever is analogous to a castle drawbridge. The chain is attached between the fulcrum and the load to raise the bridge.

Comparing Figures 15A and 15B, it is evident that Figure 15B has an indirect retainer on the first premolar, whereas Figure 15A does not. Imagine, that a piece of chewing gum is stuck to the artificial molars. What would happen if the patient opens his or her mouth? Let the load (L) be the force exerted by the chewing gum on the posterior area. In Figure 15A, the fulcrum (F, the occlusal rest on the second premolar) is located at the midpoint of the effort (E, clasp) and the load, making it a Class I lever. In other words, the clasp (which is a retainer intended to provide retention) submerges and fails to provide the initial retention.

Figure 15B shows an indirect retainer which, as the force (L) is loaded, transfers the axis of rotation to the occlusal rest on the first premolar while activating the clasp. This turns into a Class III lever, in that the effort required is larger than the load. In other words, a relatively stronger retention force (E) is required to resist the dislodging force, indicative of an inefficient lever action. Despite the inefficiency, Figure 15B represents a Kennedy Class I RPD design that properly utilizes the clasp. Now imagine altering the distance between F and E as seen in Figures 16A and 16B. With an equal force of L, it is possible to reduce the

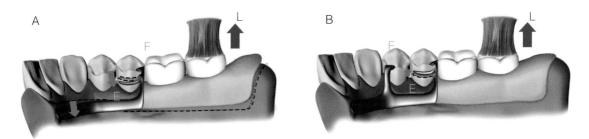

**Figure 15.** A Class III lever action that occurs with RPD movement. Figure A shows of a Class I lever action, and B shows a Class III lever action. The addition of the indirect retainer converts Class I levers into Class III levers, making the RPD more resistant to dislodging.

work done on the effort. Therefore, it is important to keep in mind how to separate the indirect retainers as far anteriorly as possible from the direct retainers.

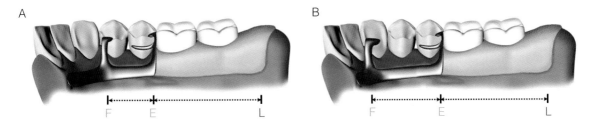

**Figure 16.** The efficiency of Class III levers relative to the location of indirect retainers. The further the indirect retainers are from the direct retainers, the more effective the function of the direct retainers.

---

**Keypoint**

**The role of indirect retainers.**

(1) They help direct retainers to dislodge in the vertical direction.

(2) They convert Class I levers into Class III levers (if the effort is on a clasp) in distal extension RPDs to provide retention.

(3) Vertical support is distributed among the additional occlusal rests.

In the Class III lever represented in Figure 15B, if we assume F is moved anteriorly, less effort (E) would be required for retention as shown in Figure 16. Understanding how stress is distributed with respect to F, E, and L is important. Indirect retainers should be placed as far away as possible from the fulcrum to maximize the efficiency of a Class III lever.

# REFERENCES

1.  Battistuzzi PG, van Slooten H, Kayser AF. Management of an anterior defect with a removable partial denture supported by implants and residual teeth: Case report. Int J Oral Maxillofac Implants 1992;7:112–115.

2.  Jang Y, Emitiaz S, Tarnow DP. Single implant-supported crown used as an abutment for a removable cast partial denture: A case report. Implant Dent 1998;7:199–204.

3.  Cecconi BT, Asgar K, Dootz E. Removable partial denture abutment tooth movement as affected by inclination of residual ridges and type of loading. J Prosthet Dent. 1971;25:375-381.

4.  Craig RG, FARAH JW. Stresses from loading distal-extension removable partial dentures. J Prosthet Dent. 1978;39:274-277.

5.  Frank RP. Direct retainers for distal-extension removable partial dentures. J Prosthet Dent. 1986;56:562-567.

6.  Ganz SD. Combination natural tooth and implant-borne removable partial denture: A clinical report. J Prosthet Dent. 1991;66:1–5.

7.  Keltjens HM, Kayser AF, Hertel R, Battistuzzi PG. Distal extension removable partial dentures supported by implants and residual teeth: Considerations and case reports. Int J Oral Maxillofac Implants 1993;8:208–213.

8.  Kihara M, Matsushita Y, Tokuhisa M, Hoshi, M, Koyano K. The effect of implant support for extended removable partial dentures–experimental studies in a model missing mandibular posterior teeth. J Jpn Soc Oral Implantol. 2003;16:214-225.

9.  Kratochvil FJ. Influence of occlusal rest position and clasp design on movement of abutment teeth. The Journal of Prosthetic Dentistry. 1963;13:114-124.

10. Luk NK, Wu VH, Liang BM, Chen Y, Yip KH, Smales RJ. Mathematical analysis of occlusal rest design for cast removable partial dentures. Eur J Prosthodont Restor Dent. 2007;15:29-32.

11. Ohkubo C, Kobayashi M, Suzuki Y, Hosoi T. Effect of implant support on distal-extension removable partial dentures: in vivo assessment. Int J Oral Maxillofac Implants. 2008;23:1095-101.

*Chapter 2-4.*

# The path of dislodgement and the path of insertion and removal must differ in RPDs

As discussed in the previous chapter, the three roles of implant or natural teeth abutments in an RPD are to provide support, stability, and retention. Among those, retention must be the last in consideration of the design, and especially, it is important to allow RPD to have minimum retention. In clinical practice, it is hard to ignore the urge to adjust the direct retainers to solve the issue of instability in unstable RPDs. Oftentimes, clasps are tightened as well. However, attempting to enhance stability may exert excessive stress on the abutment, especially on implants. There are other efficient means to prevent dislodgement of loose RPDs, such as differentiating the path of dislodgement and the path of insertion and removal of the RPD.

Retention resists vertical dislodgement of the prosthesis, and is controlled mainly by clasps (direct retainers) and adjunctively by the denture base or the surrounding soft tissues.

### Question

**A patient complains that the distal extension part of her upper RPD seems to dislodge slightly when she opens her mouth. When she chews, the denture dislodges. It appears that the degree of retention from the clasp was moderate. What could have been the problem?**

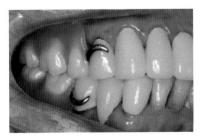 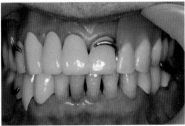 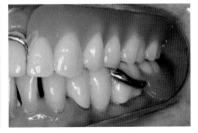

**Figure 1.** A patient experiencing dislodgement of the upper RPD upon mastication.

**Answer**

One of the reasons for such a problem could be that there are only a few remaining teeth in the anterior region. The clasp on the anterior tooth cannot be properly placed in the surveyed undercut area, resulting in insufficient retention. The lack of teeth in front of the fulcrum line also means that the indirect retainer cannot be positioned more anteriorly to improve the efficiency of the direct retainer. However, a matter of greater importance may be that the path of dislodgement of the RPD (induced by mastication) coincides with the path of insertion and removal of the RPD. If this problem is neglected in the diagnostic procedure, or the dentist is unaware of this problem, attempting to resolve this by tightening the clasps will, in turn, exert a greater amount of torsional stress on the abutment teeth (even greater in an implant).

**Keypoint**

The path of dislodgement during mastication and the path of insertion must differ in an RPD. This largely contributes to the stability of the RPD because retention is enhanced. Limiting the rotational movements caused by the Class III lever actions of distal extension RPDs is an excellent way to effectively manage RPD movements.

Surveying is also an important factor to be considered during treatment. Its purpose is to mark the proper undercut on an abutment and find the appropriate path of insertion of RPD. It is impossible to design an RPD without surveying the diagnostic cast. Some undercuts that interfere with the path of insertion and removal of RPDs may be removed.

This chapter emphasizes the importance of the path of insertion and removal indicating the appropriate retentive undercut on abutment teeth, as well as minimizing the torsional stress exerted on implant abutments.

**Question**

**What is the process of the surveying procedure? What does 'tilting of the cast' mean?**

**Answer**

The diagnostic cast is first surveyed along the horizontal plane. Placing the cast parallel to the horizontal plane presumes that the path is in line with the supposed path of dislodgement. This first step aims to find retentive undercuts along the path of dislodgement (Figure 2).

Second, the path of insertion and removal is determined by modifying the tilt of the cast from the

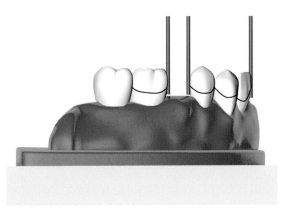

**Figure 2.** Surveying the diagnostic cast along the horizontal plane to identify retentive undercuts.

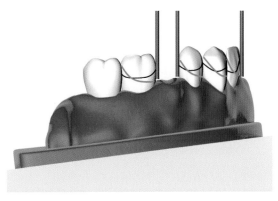

**Figure 3.** Posterior tilting. This procedure determines the path of insertion and removal and the guiding plane by modifying the tilt of the surveyor.

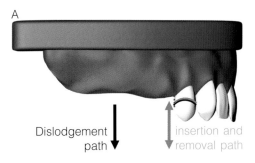

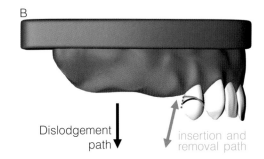

**Figure 4.** The difference between when the paths of insertion and removal and dislodgement coincide (A) and do not coincide (B). When the two paths coincide (A), the prosthesis will tend to dislodge along the path of insertion and removal, requiring stronger retention. When the two paths are different (B), proximal plates and minor connectors act to provide retention that resists the dislodging stress, providing additional stability to the prosthesis.

horizontal plane (Figure 3). As explained above, if the path of dislodgement and the path of insertion and removal coincide, the RPD will lose the stability (as well as retention) provided by the proximal plate, which guides the path of insertion and removal in one direction, and thus the RPD may experience vertical dislodging stress. In an attempt to compensate for this loss of stability, a stronger undercut engagement on the buccal aspect of the abutment teeth may be required, but it may also cause harmful stress when inserting and removing the RPD.

Generally, anterior tilting is performed for patients with posterior edentulous dentition and remaining anterior teeth, and posterior tilting is performed for patients with anterior edentulous dentition and remaining posterior teeth. This principle can be applied to both maxillary and mandibular RPDs by placing casts with teeth facing upward (as shown in Figures 2 and 3). It may be easier to imagine the

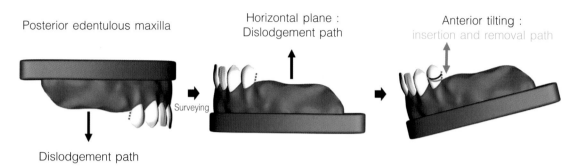

Posterior edentulous maxilla

Horizontal plane :
Dislodgement path

Anterior tilting :
insertion and removal path

Surveying

Dislodgement path

**Figure 5.** Surveying of the posterior edentulous maxilla. Additional stability can be obtained by modifying the path of insertion and removal away from the path of dislodgement. Imagine that the "heavier" side with the remaining teeth sinks down (When the guiding planes of minor connectors and proximal plates differ from the path of dislodgement, it enhances stability as well as resistance against vertical dislodging stress).

side with the remaining teeth being "heavier" and thus sinking downward. Figure 5, for instance, shows the remaining anterior teeth, anterior tilting will establish a path of insertion and removal at an acute angle with the distal surface of the abutment, with retention being provided by minor connectors (e.g., proximal plates).

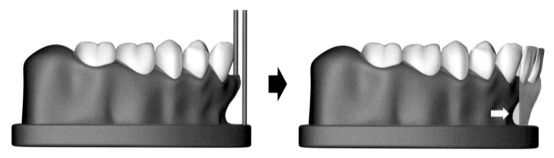

**Figure 6.** For anterior edentulous Kennedy Class IV dentition, in order to avoid potential aesthetic problems, the anterior soft tissue undercuts must be taken into consideration when determining the path of insertion.

Also, for Kennedy Class IV dentition (Figure 6), when determining the path of insertion and removal, anterior soft tissue undercuts must be considered since they may otherwise potentially result in food entrapment and unsatisfactory aesthetics.

If an anterior edentulous cast is surveyed without any tilting, a canine mesial undercut and an anterior soft tissue undercut are created. These undercuts are usually blocked out for insertion and removal when fabricating the final prosthesis, which means that the denture base would be ill-fitting on the soft tissue, and spaces would be created between the denture base and soft tissue on the buccal vestibule, ultimately resulting in unsatisfactory aesthetics.

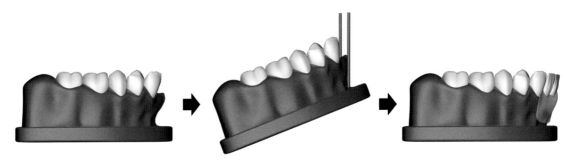

**Figure 7.** Posterior tilting allows fabrication of well-fitting and aesthetically pleasing RPDs.

This problem can be resolved by modifying the path of insertion. Posterior tilting lowers the posterior part and raises the anterior part of the denture as shown in Figure 7. Surveying at this position determines the path of insertion (whereas the path of dislodgement would be perpendicular to the occlusal plane), and this allows the parallel placement of the prosthesis without any loose gaps. Moreover, it allows the denture base to be fully engaged with the canine to compensate for the gap created by the loss of interdental papilla and/or alveolar bone.

> **Keypoint**
>
> We can minimize retentive stress on abutments by changing the path of insertion and removal from the path of dislodgement. It is important to minimize the forces of retention. As such, separating the two paths acts to prevent dislodgement not only through retentive clasps, but also through suitably designed proximal plates (minor connectors). In addition, it is important to minimize retentive undercuts on implant or natural teeth abutments. Stability cannot be compensated by retentive clasps because doing so may exert harmful torsional stress on the abutments, which is particularly true for implants.

**Question**

**How is an appropriate undercut selected when the paths of insertion and removal and the path of dislodgement differ?**

**Answer**

Since the two paths differ, the selected undercut must provide resistance against both paths.

Retentive clasp tips located in the area below the black survey line as shown in Figure 8 provide retention against denture movements perpendicular to the occlusal plane (along the path of dislodgement).

Retentive clasp tips located in the area below the blue line provide retention against movements relative to the path of insertion and removal. Therefore, the retentive clasp tips should be placed in an area where the two undercuts overlap (area C, shaded in yellow) in order to provide resistance against dislodging movements as well as provide adequate retention during insertion and removal. In this way, the function of the prosthesis can be made efficient with minimal retention forces.

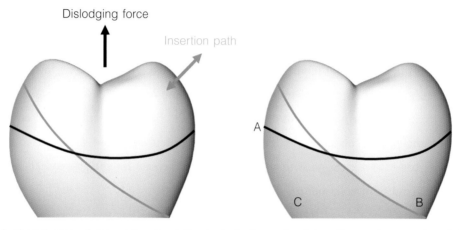

**Figure 8.** A shared area of the undercut relative to both the path of insertion and removal and the path of dislodgement must be selected. Survey line A marks the height of contour relative to the path of dislodgement. Survey line B marks the height of contour relative to the path of insertion and removal. C indicates the shared area applicable for both paths.

**Keypoint**

In the diagnostic procedure, the location of retainers must be decided upon with great deliberation. If it is difficult for the dentist to participate in the fabrication process, the dental technician should have a full understanding of these concepts, and the dentist should provide him or her with pertinent and specific feedback after intraoral assessment of the retention of the RPD. Especially for implant abutments, the dentist and the dental technician must communicate to minimize the excessive lateral force transferred to the implant abutments. As such, the goal is to fabricate ideal RPDs – particularly for implant assisted RPDs, in which abutments are more vulnerable to lateral forces.

**Is it necessary to differentiate the path of insertion and the path of dislodgement in all RPD cases?**

Answer

The previously discussed principles should be applied as much as possible where appropriate. In tooth-supported RPDs, however, sufficient retention and stability are provided by several guiding planes and retentive clasps on both ends of the edentulous area, and thus, differentiating two paths is not essential.

Distal extension RPDs have a wider range of dislodging tendencies than tooth supported RPDs. Therefore, it is essential in distal extension RPDs to modify the path of insertion by selecting an adequate tilt that allows the accommodation of efficient retention clasps.

A 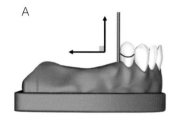 B 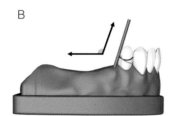 C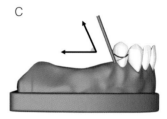

**Figure 9.** Determination of the path of insertion for distal extension RPDs. A: The path of insertion and the path of dislodgement coincide. B: The path of insertion is determined by posterior tilting. An obtuse angle is established, and consequently, more frequent denture movements can be expected. C: The path of insertion is determined by anterior tilting. An acute angle is established, and this will help minor connectors confine denture movements. (Note: Tilting is exaggerated in the diagram for a better visual explanation. Tilting must not be excessive in real practice.)

Surveying at an angle parallel to the direction of dislodgement (as in Figure 9A) tends to cause the prosthesis dislodge in the same direction with insertion path during mastication. If the cast is raised anteriorly to be surveyed (also known as posterior tilting), the dislodging angle is established at an obtuse angle, and a wider range of angles of dislodgement are rendered. On the other hand, if the cast is raised posteriorly (also known as anterior tilting) relative to the path of insertion and removal, a smaller range of angles of dislodgement would be rendered. More importantly, the minor connector (e.g. proximal plate) is then placed on the distal inclination of the abutment, confining the rotational movements of the distal extension of the RPD as well as of the prosthesis itself.

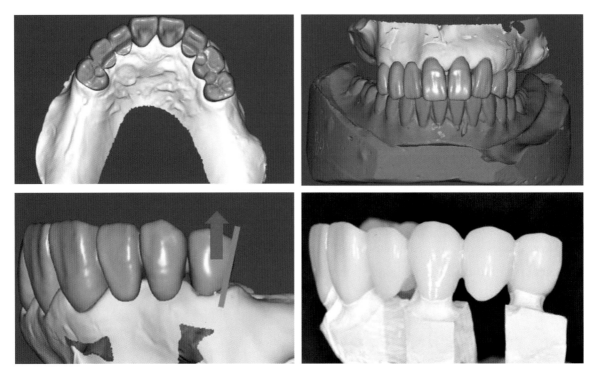

**Figure 10.** Determination of the path of dislodgement (red arrow) and the path of insertion and removal (blue line). Intentionally selecting a path of insertion and removal that is different from the path of dislodgement will allow confinement of rotational movements from the distal extension and increase the stability of the RPD. It is important to make sure the direction of insertion for all the proximal plates and all the minor connectors connecting the rests, are parallel to one another.

> **Keypoint**
>
> In order to minimize the biomechanical problems mentioned in the first section of this chapter, it is important to anteriorly tilt the cast and establish the distal undercut on the abutment at acute angles (this determines resistance against the vertical dislodging force). If the circumstances are not favorable for intraoral tooth preparation, a surveyed crown restoration is recommended.

# REFERENCES

1. Bezzon OL, MATTOS MGC, RIBERO RF. Surveying removable partial dentures: the importance of guiding planes and path of insertion for stability. The Journal of prosthetic dentistry, 1997;78:412-418.

2. Bohnenkamp DM. Removable partial dentures: clinical concepts. Dental Clinics of North America. 2014;58:69-89.

3. Chrystie JA. Principles of clasp retention: a review. Aust Dent J. 1988;33:96-100.

4. Coy RE, ARNOLD PD. Survey and design of diagnostic casts for removable partial dentures. The Journal of prosthetic dentistry. 1974;32:103-106.

5. Davenport J, Basker RM, Heath JR, Ralph JP, Glantz PO. Surveying. British dental journal. 2000;189:532-542.

6. Johnson DL. Adapting a dental surveyor to function in two planes. J Prosthodont. 1993;2:206-210.

7. Stern WJ. Guiding planes in clasp reciprocation and retention. The Journal of prosthetic dentistry. 1975;34:408-414.

8. Stratton RJ, Wiebelt FJ. Surveying in removable partial denture design. Quintessence Dent Technol. 1984;8:237-242.

*Chapter 2-5.*

# Cantilever support can be harmful to RPD abutments, especially to implant abutments

**Question**

## What is cantilever support?

**Answer**

Cantilever support is also known as indirect support. Indirect retention helps to obtain effective retention by making direct retainers disengage vertically. In other words, it acts as a hard wall (in the form of rests or a hard palate) located anterior to a fulcrum line that is formed when an RPD is about to dislodge. This enables the direct retainer to work efficiently. Similarly, indirect support aids RPDs by supporting

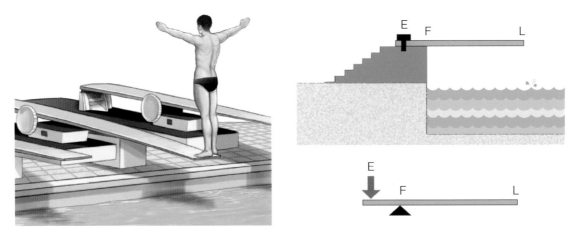

**Figure 1.** Example of cantilever support. The diving board works as a Class I leverage and is firmly held at point E, which allows divers to jump at point L.

areas that lack support. However, if the cantilever support is incorrectly designed, it can be harmful to abutments, especially to implant abutments because it may apply an excessive lateral force.

It appears that Class I levers have more intraoral disadvantages than advantages (see Chapter 2.3). Figure 1 shows a diver diving from a board, illustrating the act of a Class I lever.

The diving board does not have any vertical support. When jumping from point L, a rotational axis is formed at point F, and the fixed pins at point E support the board. The function of point E is to offer indirect support or cantilever support. If there were to be a solid wall under point L, it would act as direct support. Without such direct support, the fixed pins at point E play a role in maintaining support. If they become weak, the diver could fall.

### Question

**Cantilever support can exert harmful forces on the abutments embraced with clasps located anterior to the rotational axis. When do we need this kind of support for RPDs?**

### Answer

Theoretically, cantilever support can exert undesired forces onto the abutments. However, as previously mentioned, it can be advantageous in some cases.

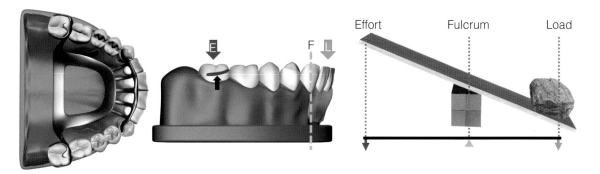

**Figure 2.** A case in which cantilever support in a Kennedy Class IV RPD is advantageous.

The Kennedy Class IV patient is missing four anterior teeth (Figure 2). In order to compensate for alveolar bone absorption and the four missing anterior teeth, creating an RPD can be a valid treatment option. Let's assume that the patient is having a bite of pizza with the anterior part of the RPD. Because there is alveolar bone absorption under the four anterior teeth, rotation will occur around both cingulum rests. What prevents this rotation are the clasps located on the undercuts of both second molars.

Therefore, the clasps located on the second molars offer cantilever or indirect support to prevent the rotation of the RPD. The clasps that provide indirect support must have sufficient retention to withstand the rotation of the RPD. The abutments, teeth, or implants should also be strong enough to provide cantilever support. If such factors are not taken into account, the clasps may be easily fractured and the abutments become more prone to damage. However, utilizing cantilever support is unavoidable with RPDs, so the aforementioned must be seriously considered.

> **Keypoint**
>
> When planning to utilize cantilever support, the mechanisms of the Class I lever must be well understood. In this type of lever, the stress is more efficiently dispersed as the distance between the fulcrum (F) and the point of resistance by the clasps (E) is increased; as the E-F distance increases, the strength required from (E) to withstand load (L) is decreased.

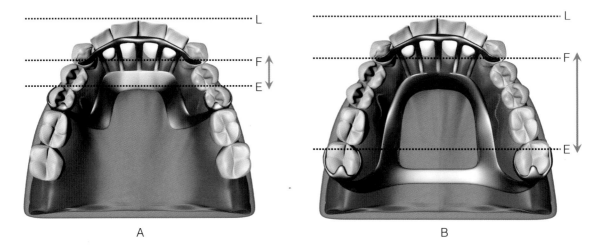

**Figure 3.** The varying efficiencies of cantilever support according to the distance between the fulcrum (F) and the point of resistance by the clasps (E).

Imagine designing an RPD to replace four missing anterior teeth, as shown in Figure 3. When comparing the two cases shown, the distance between point F (fulcrum line, rotational axis) and E (resistance point of the clasps) is different. Even though they are both Class I levers, as the distance between point F and E increases, the force at point E resisting the force exerted at point L decreases. Also, when the same force is exerted at point E in both cases, a greater force is needed at point L as seen in Figure B in order to dislodge the clasps. Thus, it is evident that with a thorough understanding of Class I lever actions, the force transmitted to the abutments can be minimized and the efficiency of the cantilever support can be simultaneously maximized.

### Question

**What is the difference between the two designs for Kennedy Class IV RPDs in the figure below, and which one is better?**

### Answer

Figures 4A and B are not very different in terms of cantilever support because the distance between points E and F are roughly the same. However, the clasp coming from the distal area of the upper second molar is more efficient in terms of retention. If both clasps are located in the proper undercut, the clasps will offer a similar amount of cantilever support when biting with incisors. Imagine biting down on sticky food with anterior teeth. When opening the mouth, the RPD tends to dislodge. When this happens, the rotational axis becomes the line connecting the two rests on both second molars. As shown in Figure

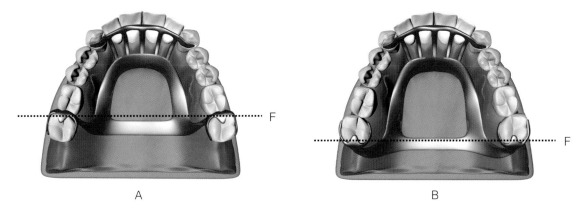

A                    B

**Figure 4.** Clasp assemblies can function differently, even when located on the same teeth, depending on how they are positioned.

5A, when the RPD dislodges, the tip of the clasps moves apically along the rotational axis. Though the amount of movement is not that significant, the retentive role of the clasp is not properly fulfilled. In contrast, as seen in Figure 5B, when the RPD dislodges, the rotational axis becomes the line that connects the distal rests on both second molars, and the tip of the clasps located anterior to the rotational axis resists against dislodgement by providing retention. In other words, if the RPD dislodges, A will display a Class I lever action, and B will display a Class III lever action, having the clasps act as effort points.

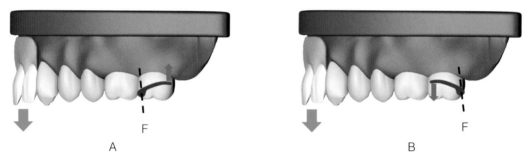

A          B

**Figure 5.** When the anterior portion of the RPD dislodges vertically, the clasps in A and B function differently based on their placement.

As shown in Figure 5, case B is superior to case A in resisting RPD dislodgement. However, this is not always true. It must be kept in mind that the path of dislodgement and the path of insertion and removal must differ (see Chapter 2.4).

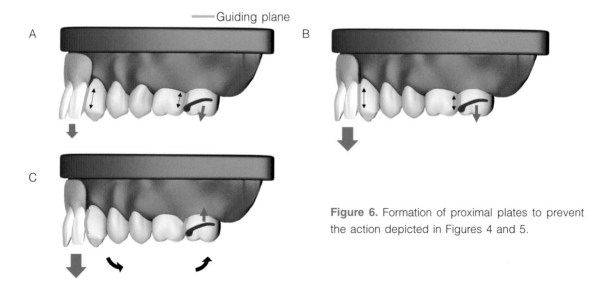

Guiding plane

A

B

C

**Figure 6.** Formation of proximal plates to prevent the action depicted in Figures 4 and 5.

As shown in Figure 6, the path of insertion and removal, which is different from the path of dislodgement, is formed on the mesial of the canine and the interproximal space of the second molars by surveying with posterior tilting. Through this, when the RPD is about to dislodge, the rotational movement does not occur (Figure 6A). In addition, the clasps located on the second molars resist against the RPD's dislodging force, which occurs along the path of insertion and removal. As seen in Figure 6B, the path of insertion and removal coincides with the path of dislodgement, and thus greater retention from the clasp is needed to resist the dislodgement (Figure 6B). Nevertheless, due to the proximal plates, the rotational movement can still be minimized. Even so, the RPD dislodges more easily in case B than in case A. Now, consider Figure 6C. If the path of insertion and removal is formed without surveying, the path of dislodgement is widened, the RPD rotates around the mesial rests of the second molars, and the clasps move apically. In other words, the clasps do not provide initial retention. This type of RPD has little stability and has great mobility.

---

**Keypoint**

(1) Implants acting as RPD abutments have less mobility and elasticity than natural teeth. Therefore, extra care should be taken to avoid transfer of harmful forces to the implant abutments.

(2) An RPD metal framework should be designed efficiently to evenly distribute the forces among, and minimize damage done to, the abutments. But if this cannot be achieved through the design, accurate impressions (e.g. functional impression) and fabricating a well-fitting denture base minimize the rotational movements. If this is still not enough, establish a bilaterally balanced occlusion. Overall, if implants are being used as abutments, and the number of abutments is small, the RPD's design, impression, and occlusal scheme must be considered in order to establish stability.

---

**Question**

## Under what conditions does cantilever support exert harmful forces to abutments?

**Answer**

It is important to remember that if an RPD has little to no movement, or if an abutment that is provided with cantilever support is strong enough to withstand such movement, the risk of using cantilever support is reduced.

Think about the clasp that holds the upper right first premolar in Figure 7A. If the edentulous tissue is not firm, movement of the RPD during mastication can be anticipated. Since the clasp on the upper right first premolar is located anterior to the fulcrum line (F), this movement may exert extrusive forces

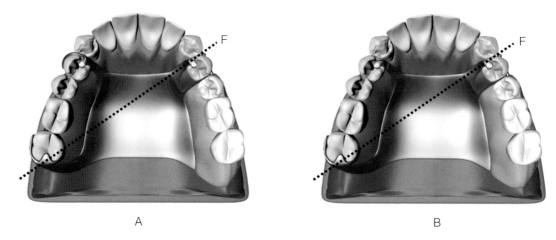

A                                                                    B

**Figure 7.** Understanding the difference in the designs of two Kennedy Class II RPDs.

onto the tooth via the clasp every time the patient masticates. This is an example of improper usage of cantilever support. An important point here is that if an accurate impression is taken of the edentulous area via a functional impression, the RPD movement will be reduced. In this case, the clasp can be placed on the upper right first premolar at the dentist's discretion, and it may not cause such harmful stress on the abutment. Placing only a rest on the upper right first premolar is another feasible option, which is presented in Figure 7B. If the goal of treatment is to provide minimal retention, the clasps on the upper right second molar and the upper left first premolar might be just enough. The rest on the upper right first premolar acts as an indirect retainer and can also provide vertical support to the RPD.

Though it is possible that the direct retainer on the upper right second molar may extrude the tooth, that type of movement is unlikely here because molars are relatively strong abutments and also because there is additional support from the palate, as well as additional stability from the minor connectors. If an RPD is made properly, it will have little to no movement.

## Question

**What factors should be considered when designing implant-assisted RPDs with two implant abutments (surveyed prostheses) as shown in Figure 8?**

## Answer

First, in Figure 8A, implants are placed in the upper right second molar and the upper left second

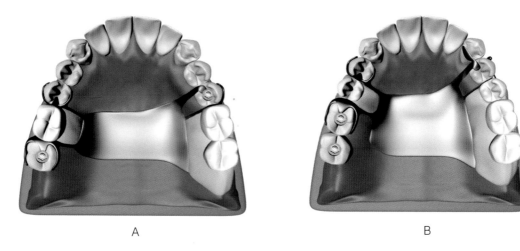

A              B

**Figure 8.** Designing cantilever support when using implants as abutments.

premolar area. In this case, we can assume that the remaining teeth are in good condition without any pathology. In this Kennedy Class II modification I RPD, an indirect retainer is formed anterior to the fulcrum line connecting the rests on the upper right second molar and the upper left second premolar. A rest on the upper right second premolar functions as the indirect retainer. However, the clasp on that tooth is harmful, as it can also act as a cantilever. The upper right molar area is tooth-supported and the upper left molar area is missing only two molars. There are three rests on the upper right second molar, second premolar, and left second premolar. There are also four proximal plates on the mesial to the upper right second molar, distal to the upper right second premolar, and mesial and distal to the upper left second premolar. Taken together then, because most of the movement of the RPD is stabilized by the abutments, harmful forces exerted on the upper right second premolar from cantilever support is considered negligible. If the dentist so desires, the clasp can be placed. If the dentist is concerned about the harmful forces transferred to the implant abutments, the clasp can be exchanged for a wrought wire or can be eliminated entirely. In the maxilla, splinting two or more implants, as shown in Figure 8B, is recommended.

> **Keypoint**
>
> There is no single correct RPD design. The treatment plan should be decided based on an understanding of the possible movements of RPD. However, there are various problems that may arise such as denture fractures and damage to abutments (especially to implant abutments). Therefore, the RPD should be designed with careful consideration. Fabrication of implant-assisted RPDs for maximized efficiency requires a solid understanding of the basic principles of RPD fabrication.

# REFERENCES

1. Avant WE. Indirect retention in partial denture design. J Prosthet Dent. 2003;90:1-5.

2. Ben-Ur Z, Aviv I, Maharshak B. Factors affecting displacement of free-end saddle removable partial dentures. Quintessence Int. 1991;22:23-7.

3. Bezzon OL, Mattos MGC, Ribeiro RF. Surveying removable partial dentures: the importance of guiding planes and path of insertion for stability. J Prosthet Dent. 1997;78:412-418.

4. Bezzon OL, Ribeiro RF, Pagnano VO. Device for recording the path of insertion for removable partial dentures. J Prosthet Dent. 2000;84:136-138.

5. Clark RK, Chow TW. A reappraisal of indirect retention in removable partial dentures with long bilateral distal-extension saddles. Quintessence Int. 1995;26:253-255.

6. Frank RP, Nicholls JI. An investigation of the effectiveness of indirect retainers. J Prosthet Dent. 1977;38:494-506.

7. LaVere AM clasp retention: the effects of five variables. J Prosthodont. 1993;2:126-131.

8. Mijiritsky E. Implants in conjunction with removable partial dentures: a literature review. Implant Dent. 2007;16:146-54.

9. Preston KP. The bilateral distal extension removable partial denture: mechanical problems and solutions. Eur J Prosthodont Restor Dent. 2007;15:115-121.

10. Stern WJ. Guiding planes in clasp reciprocation and retention. J Prosthet Dent. 1975;34:408-414.

# Understanding the stability of an implant-assisted RPD is crucial to its success

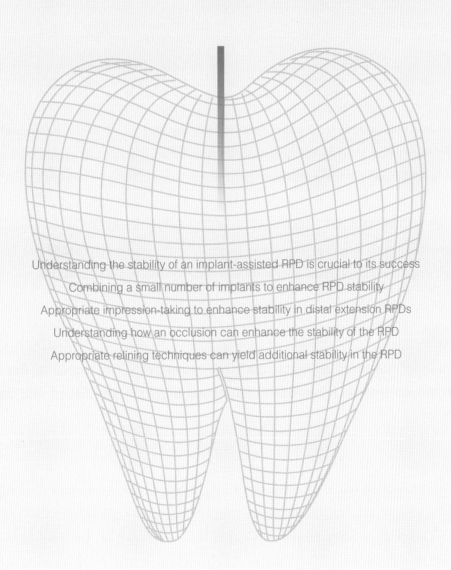

Chapter 3-1.

# Understanding the stability of an implant-assisted RPD is crucial to its success

Chapter 3 will first investigate how to prevent movements that may occur in the tooth- and tissue-supported RPDs, and second, describe the design of RPDs in detail using a small number of implants. Again, it should be noted that the abutments mentioned throughout the book include both natural teeth and implants.

This chapter will provide in-depth explanations on the design of the RPD, the impression-taking methods, the occlusal scheme, as well as the relining processes to ensure the support and stability of the RPD. A thorough understanding of this chapter will aid in better comprehension of the chapters to follow.

## Question

**It was mentioned that three different rotational movements can occur in the RPDs. Would such movements be minimized if additional implants are placed and used as abutments?**

## Answer

There is no single definite answer to this question; it is up to the dentists to use their discretion.

As shown in Figure 1, three rotational movements can occur in the RPDs. The first is a rotational movement around the fulcrum line passing through the posterior most part of the abutment, in which the denture base moves vertically toward or away from the supporting residual ridge. This tissue-ward movement is common in distal extension RPDs. The second is a rotational movement around the

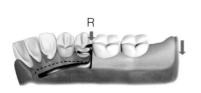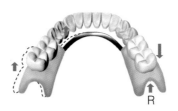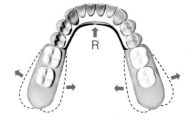

**Figure 1.** Three different rotational movements may occur in the RPDs.

longitudinal axis formed by the crest of the residual ridge. This movement can occur when bite force is applied to artificial teeth that are located buccal to the alveolar ridge due to severe bone resorption. The third is a rotational movement around the vertical axis located near the center of the arch. Usually, this occurs when there are only a few abutments, when there are not enough guiding planes, or when the denture lacks adequate stabilization.

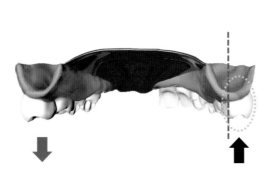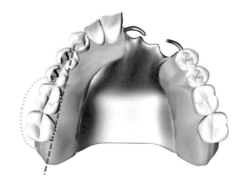

**Figure 2.** Rotational movements that may occur when an occlusal force is applied on the artificial teeth located buccal to the alveolar ridge. This is a situation in which the number of remaining abutments is small and buccal alveolar bone resorption is severe (Red line: location of alveolar ridge).

The second aforementioned movement is displayed in Figure 2. When the buccal alveolar bone of the edentulous area is severely resorbed, the artificial teeth (circled in yellow) are positioned further outward than the alveolar ridge (indicated by the red line). In this case, when an occlusal force is applied to the artificial teeth, a Class I lever action takes place, lifting the left side of the denture. This rotational movement may not be a major problem if the abutment is properly positioned to prevent any rotation, but if the abutment is unable to prevent such rotation, it can be prevented by creating a bilateral balanced occlusion or an intentional posterior crossbite occlusion (see Chapter 3.4).

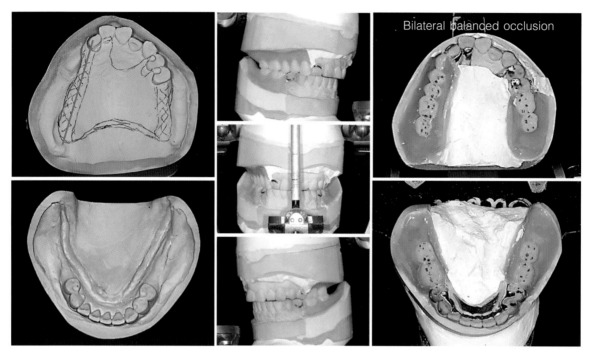

**Figure 3.** Bilateral balanced occlusion can reduce a rotation of the denture, predicted by severe buccal alveolar bone resorption in the maxilla.

A stable RPD can resist these rotational movements. Stability is enhanced by proper positioning and a greater number of abutments.

As shown in Figure 4A, if healthy abutments are sufficiently present, a tooth-supported RPD design can be used, and the guiding planes parallel to the path of RPD insertion can be formed on the proximal surface of the four abutments. The reciprocal arm can be placed on the lingual surface of the abutment, and the minor connector (add the proximal plate) that connects these clasps can prevent the previously mentioned, undesired

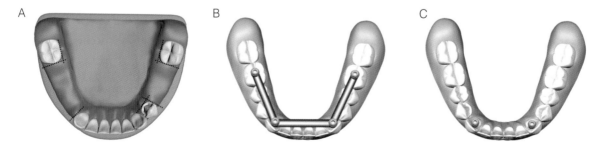

**Figure 4.** The stability of RPDs is determined by the number of abutments (natural teeth or implants).

movements. In a fully edentulous patient, four implants can be placed to make an overdenture as shown in Figure 4B, to mimic the effect of a tooth-supported RPD, in which all potential movements are prevented by the four implants. However, it should be noted that even if the bar is created on the four implants, denture movement may still occur, as in tooth- and tissue-supported RPDs. This will be further explained in Chapter 4. On the other hand, if the two implants are placed as shown in Figure 4C, a rotational axis connecting these two implants will be formed, as in a distal extension RPD.

> **Keypoint**
>
> Even with implant-assisted RPDs, there is a possibility that movements may still occur. The harmful lateral force created by these movements may transfer directly to the abutments (especially if the implant itself is the abutment). It is therefore important to ensure sufficient stability of the RPD itself to minimize rotational movements.

Even with four solitary type attachments (Figure 5B), the stability of the implant is no different from that of the one with two attachments (Figure 5A). The two additional attachments only enhance retention. On the other hand, if the attachments are placed at a distance in the anterior-posterior direction (A-P spread), stability would be increased (Figure 5C); thereby, increasing the area of the hard wall and reducing the likelihood of denture movements.

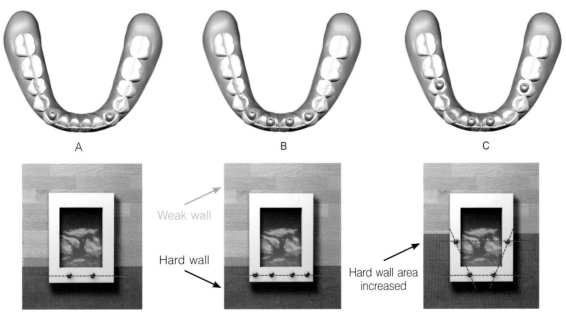

**Figure 5.** A comparison of the varying stability of overdentures as determined by the number and location of implants.

> **Keypoint**
>
> The number of implants does not necessarily correlate with the stability of an RPD. The appropriate number and proper positioning of the implants determine the stability.

**Question**

### Which are the factors that must be taken into consideration when designing an RPD that is not fully supported and stabilized by abutments?

**Answer**

RPDs that are not firmly held by abutments inevitably generate rotational movements. If these movements are strongly blocked, excessive force is transferred to the abutments instead, rather than being balanced across both the abutments as well as the residual ridge. It is therefore important to minimize the lateral or rotational force exerted on the abutments.

As shown in Figure 6, in a tooth-supported RPD, vertical tissue-ward movements can be sufficiently prevented if the rests are properly formed. However, in a distal extension RPD, vertical rotational movements around the fulcrum line of the posterior-most abutments cannot be avoided. Among the three previously mentioned types of movements, the upward and downward rotational movement around the fulcrum line may be prevented with an appropriately designed RPD.

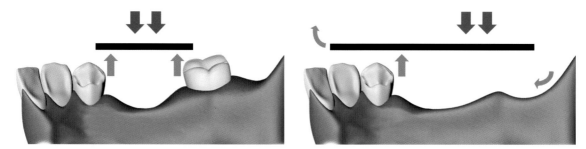

**Figure 6.** Movements that occur in the tooth-supported RPD and the tooth- and tissue-supported RPD (distal extension RPD). To minimize the force generated by the rotation of a distal extension RPD on the abutments, a direct retainer that allows functional vertical movement of the RPD and an indirect retainer that aids the function of the direct retainer are required.

Key Takeaway: With a distal extension RPD, both an indirect retainer and a direct retainer of stress breaker type are needed to relieve the stress on abutments

To minimize the force generated by the rotational movement on the abutments, a direct retainer (RPI, RPA, wrought wire etc.) should be added to relieve stress and allow for functional movement of the RPD, and an indirect retainer can be added to help the direct retainer function vertically.

## Question

**What are the factors that should be taken into consideration to minimize tissue-ward movement of the denture base?**

## Answer

The factors to be taken into consideration to minimize the tissue-ward movement of the RPDs are as follows.

(1) Rests with an appropriate shape and position.

(2) Major and minor connectors that have sufficient strength.

(3) An even distribution of forces to the edentulous alveolar ridge that can be achieved by sufficiently extending the denture base and taking functional impressions as necessary.

(4) Movement control through occlusal considerations when there are not enough abutments.

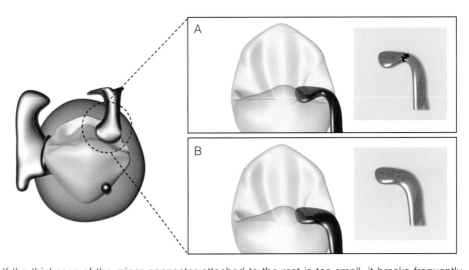

**Figure 7.** If the thickness of the minor connector attached to the rest is too small, it breaks frequently.

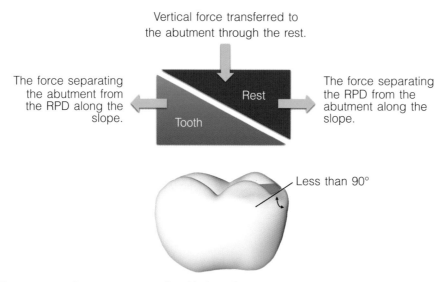

**Figure 8.** The rest must form an acute angle with the minor connector to generate an occlusal force along the long axis. Obtuse angles cause sliding movements, which increase the horizontal force acting upon the abutment.

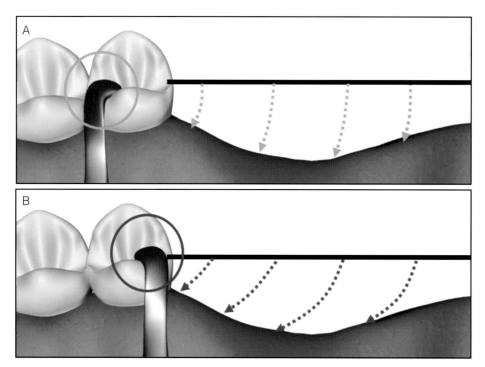

**Figure 9.** Various rest positions of the posterior-most abutment in a distal extension RPD.
Here, it is better to place the occlusal rest of the posterior-most abutment mesially (A) than distally (B). A mesially located occlusal rest may exert a more vertical force towards the residual ridge given the larger diameter of rotational movement around the fulcrum line.

There are two important considerations regarding the proper positioning and shape of the rest. First, the rest and the minor connector attached to the rest need to be strong enough to withstand vertical occlusal forces. The minimum thickness of the minor connector should be between 1.0 and 1.5 mm, as shown in Figure 7. Additionally, the rest connected to the minor connectors should form an acute angle, or a lateral force will be exerted upon the abutment following the exertion of an occlusal force, as shown in Figure 8.

Second, in a distal extension RPD, the occlusal rest of the abutment adjacent to the edentulous area should be positioned mesially to transfer a more vertical occlusal force to the residual ridge (Figure 9).

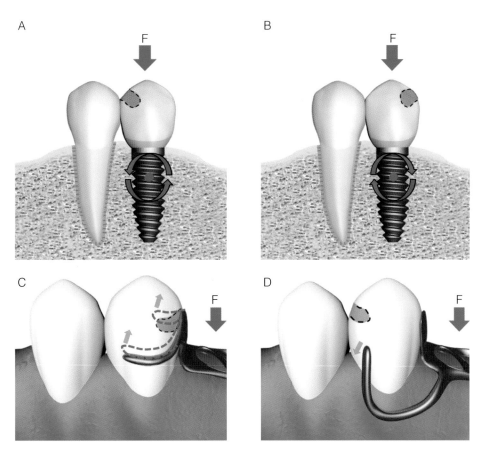

**Figure 10.** Benefits of a mesial rest with a distal extension RPD. As shown in (A), a rotational force acting counterclockwise on the abutment tooth transfers the stress to the anteriorly positioned residual tooth. Conversely, if the distal rest is formed as shown in (B), a clockwise rotational force moves the abutment distally. Also with a mesial rest, the clasp can immediately move away from the abutment during a tissue-ward movement thereby reducing the external force on the abutment (D). However, with a distal rest as shown in (C), the clasp can produce a Class I lever action following a tissue-ward movement of distal extension denture base.

Additionally, if an occlusal force is exerted on a distally positioned abutment, the anteriorly positioned clasp may act as a Class I lever, extruding the abutment. However, with a mesial rest, the clasp is positioned posterior to the rest, and the clasp tip moves in the same direction as that of the RPD rotation, minimizing the harmful forces exerted upon the abutment. These clasps are referred to as stress breakers that can accommodate the functional movements of the RPD.

## Question

**Despite precautionary measures, there may be cases in which the tissue-ward movement of a distal extension RPD is inevitable. What are the key features that need to be taken into consideration to design an RPD that will not damage the abutment even with a tissue-ward movement?**

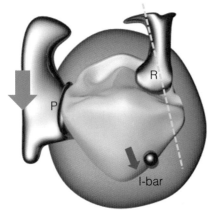

R=Mesial Rest
P=Distal Guiding Plate
I=I-shaped Retentive Clasp
A=Arm-shaped Retentive Clasp

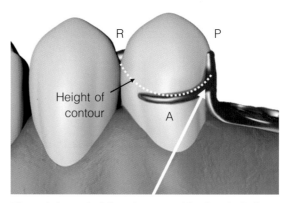

The origin part of the clasp must be located along the height of the contour or must be sufficiently relieved.

**Figure 11** Comparison of the RPI and RPA systems. Both utilize a mesial rest, and since there is no reciprocal arm, the proximal plate extends slightly onto the lingual surface of the abutment for enhanced stability. When the occlusal force is exerted on the edentulous area, it generates a slight rotation centered around the mesial rest, which then makes the I-bar move downward and forward, preventing the transfer of forces onto the abutment. In an RPA system, the origin part of the clasp must be located along the height of the contour or be sufficiently relieved, so that it does not interfere with rotational movements. Otherwise, with slight rotational movements, the origin part of the clasp comes in contact with the vertical part of the contour on the abutment tooth. This contact point becomes the new rotational axis, lifting the mesial rest. The clasp then extrudes the abutment. The dentist must keep this in mind when trying different metal frameworks.

> **Answer**

As previously mentioned, it is important to protect the abutment by designing a clasp that can accommodate functional movements with a distal extension RPD. These clasp designs include RPIs, RPAs, and wrought wire clasps.

The RPI or RPA systems minimize the force exerted on the abutment through the shape of the clasp assembly, and the wrought wire clasps reduce the force transferred to the abutment because of its physical properties such as high elasticity. The RPI system consists of a clasp assembled with a mesial rest, proximal plate, and an I-bar, and the RPA system uses Akers instead of the I-bar. Although the functional principles of both the clasps are the same, the RPA system is used when tissue undercuts are severe or space is insufficient to implement the I-bar (i.e. when the vestibule is shallow). The placement of the rest, clasp, and proximal plate in an RPI system will determine whether the forces exerted upon a distal extension RPD during mastication will be transferred to the abutment or to the residual ridge. There are three different combinations created by Kratochvil (1963), Krol (1973), and Demer (1976). There is no single best option, therefore the condition of the abutment should be taken into consideration before making a judgment.

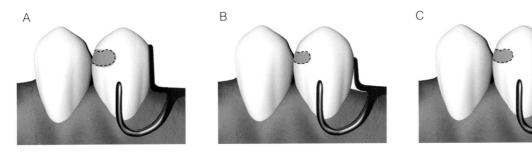

**Figure 12.** Varying designs of the RPI system.

A. A large, definite rest is formed with the guiding plane close to the gingiva. The proximal plate is in full contact with no space in between. In this case, all the horizontal force generated by tissue-ward movements of the RPD is directly transferred to the abutment. If the abutment is sound, or if multiple implants are splinted to form the abutment, this design is appropriate.

B. A small rest and a 2-3 mm long guiding plane is formed, with 1/3 of the surface in contact with the clasp. About 1 mm of the proximal plate is in contact, so when a masticatory pressure is applied, the proximal plate immediately slides into the proximal undercut. This allows for maximum movement of the RPD and maximum transfer of the occlusal force to the residual alveolar ridge.

C. This is most widely applied in clinical practices. The resulting movement of the RPD in C is in between those of A and B.

The problem with Figure 12B is indicated in Figure 13; the proximal plate falls off from the abutment immediately following a tissue-ward movement by the RPD. In this case, the proximal plate is pushed downward and the clasp tip comes in contact with the abutment. This forms a Class 1 lever, lifting the rest upward. In other words, it becomes significantly more unstable, and harmful external forces may be

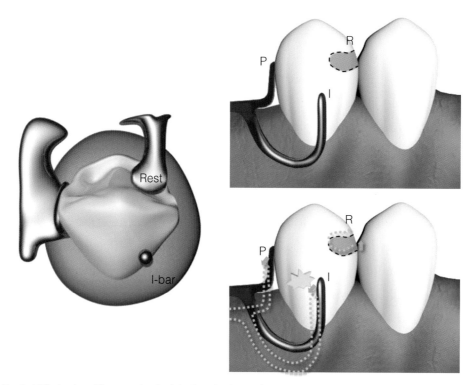

**Figure 13** Krol's RPI design. The proximal plate has both a minor connector and a stabilizing factor, and should always be in contact with the abutment during insertion and removal of the RPD. Here, the proximal plate may fall off from the abutment immediately following a tissue-ward movement by the RPD, and the clasp tip contacting with the abutment may form a new rotational axis.

exerted on the abutment. Given that the proximal plate is a minor connector contributing to the stability of the RPD, the proximal plate should always be in contact with the abutment, both during insertion, as well as during functional movements, so that all the components of the RPD can function properly.

Kratochvil's design has the potential to transfer excessive lateral force onto the abutment, while Krol's design has the potential to lose its stability; therefore, Demer's design is the most appropriate to be implemented when designing RPI and RPA (Figure 14).

Another factor to consider when designing an RPI system is whether it allows for some mesial movement by the minor connector attached to the mesial rest (Figure 15).

One last factor to be taken into consideration is regarding the positioning of the I-bar. As shown in Figure 16, the recommendation is to place the I-bar between points B and C.

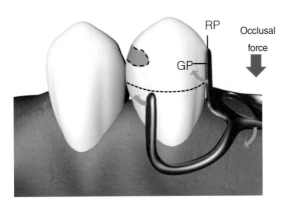

**Figure 14.** Demer's design. The guiding plane extends from the distal marginal ridge of the abutment to the junction between the middle third and cervical third. The proximal plate is in contact with the entire surface of the guiding plane. This allows for some rotational movement during mastication, which ensures that the occlusal force is evenly distributed to the abutment and the residual ridge. The key point here is that the proximal plate should never fall off from the guiding plane during RPD movements of any kind.

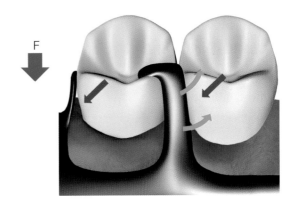

**Figure 15.** Lingual view of the minor connector attached to the mesial rest in an RPI system. When the RPD undergoes a tissue-ward movement, the minor connector moves forward and upward. If the mesial surface of the minor connector is in complete contact with the teeth, it will interfere with such movements and exert a horizontal force on the anterior tooth. If the two teeth are not splinted, there is the possibility of creating unwanted space between the teeth or damaging the adjacent tooth. Additionally, the minor connector may be fractured during mastication.

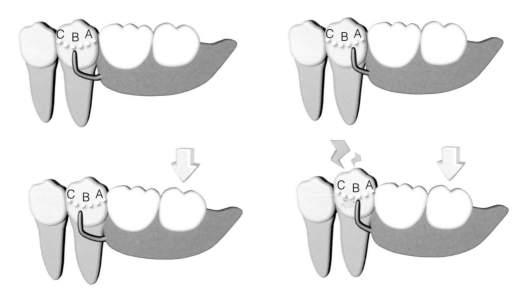

**Figure 16.** An appropriate placement of the I-bar in an RPI system allows for tissue-ward movements by the RPD. During such movements, the clasp may also undergo a slight movement in either the anterior-inferior or anterior-superior direction. If the I-bar is located at point A, it will produce an unwanted force on the abutment during mastication. Therefore, the I-bar should be placed between B and C. However, it should be noted that if the I-bar is located too close to point C, it may generate a Class I lever action, producing a pulling force on the abutment because it is positioned more anteriorly from the rest.

## Question

**Can the safety of the abutment (either tooth or implant) during movements by a distal extension RPD be guaranteed if the RPI or RPA system is placed on the posterior most abutment?**

## Answer

There is no such guarantee. While the design of the RPI or RPA system itself can reduce the amount of undesired force transferred to the abutment, the positioning of the clasp is just as important (see Figure 17,18 and 19).

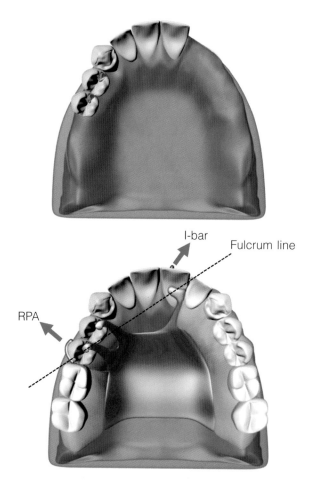

**Figure 17.** An RPD with the upper right 2nd premolar and upper left central incisor serving as abutments. Upper right 2nd premolar and upper left central incisor are designed with an RPA and I-Bar, respectively, allowing for some RPD movement. The I-bar and RPA move in a direction that extrudes the abutment when the RPD undergoes tissue-ward movements around the fulcrum line.

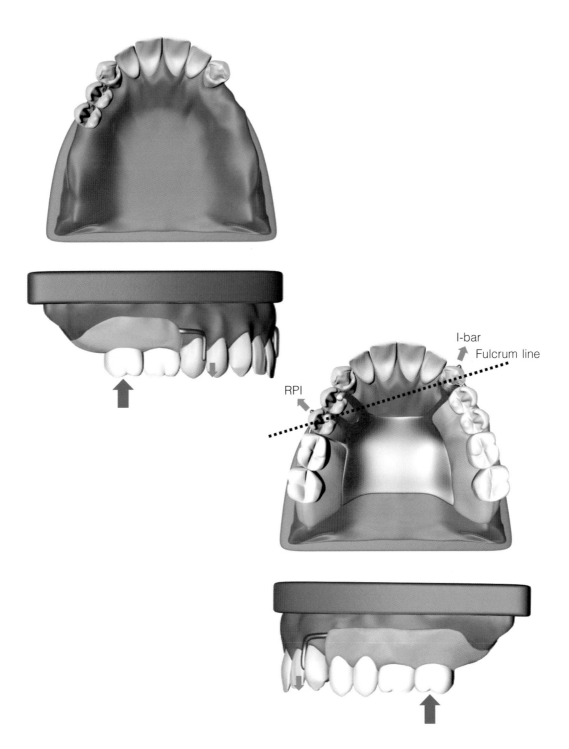

**Figure 18.** An RPD with the upper right 2nd premolar and the upper left canine serving as abutments. Upper left lateral incisor and canine have been added from Figure 17. In this case, the I-bars on the upper left canine and upper right 2nd premolar are located anterior to the fulcrum line, which causes Class I lever action, similar to what is shown in Figure 17. This creates the possibility that the I-bar extrudes the abutment teeth during mastication.

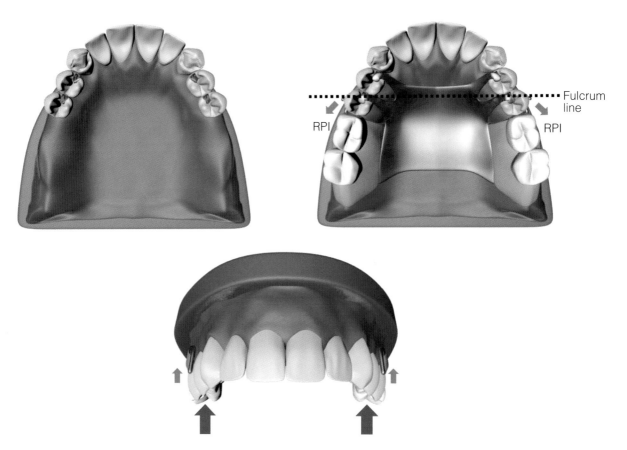

**Figure 19.** RPD design with the upper left 2nd premolar and upper right 2nd premolar serving as abutments. In this case, the clasp is located on or posterior to the fulcrum line, creating a true RPI system that can allow a certain degree of movement during a tissue-ward movement by the RPD.

**Keypoint**

We should be able to image the rotational movement around the rests on the most posterior abutments by displacement of free- end saddle RPD.

However, if it is difficult to design an RPD that allows for tissue-ward movements like Figure 17 and 18, a wrought wire clasp could be used. Additionally, denture movement can be minimized by taking a functional impression of the posterior edentulous area and creating a bilaterally balanced occlusion.

As shown in Figure 17, 18, and 19, RPI or RPA direct retainers, which allow for tissue-ward movements by the RPD, should be located symmetrically, and should only be implemented if premolars are present.

# REFERENCES

1.  Avant WE. Fulcrum and retention lines in planning removable partial dentures. J Prosthet Dent. 1971;25:162-166.

2.  Ben-Ur Z1, Aviv I, Maharshak B. Factors affecting displacement of free-end saddle removable partial dentures. Quintessence Int. 1991;22:23-27.

3.  Cecconi BT. Effect of rest design on transmission of forces to abutment teeth. J Prosthet Dent. 1974;32:141-151.

4.  Clark RK1, Chow TW. A reappraisal of indirect retention in removable partial dentures with long bilateral distal-extension saddles. Quintessence Int. 1995;26:253-255.

5.  Craig RG, Farah JW. Stresses from loading distal-extension removable partial dentures. J Prosthet Dent. 1978;39:274-277.

6.  De Aquino AR, Barreto AO, de Aquino LM, Ferreira ÂM, Carreiro Ada FJ, Longitudinal clinical evaluation of undercut areas and rest seats of abutment teeth in removable partial denture treatment. J Prosthodont. 2011;20:639-642.

7.  Demer WJ. An analysis of mesial rest-I-bar clasp designs. J Prosthet Dent. 1976;36:243-253.

8.  Eliason CM. RPA clasp design for distal-extension removable partial dentures. J Prosthet Dent. 1983;49:25-27.

9.  Jensen C, Meijer HJA, Raghoebar GM, Kerdijk W, Cune MS. Implant-supported removable partial dentures in the mandible: A 3-16 year retrospective study. 5 J Prosthodont Res. 2017;61:98-105.

10. Kotowicz WE, Fisher RL, Reed RA, Jaslow C. The combination clasp and the distal extension removable partial denture. Dent Clin North Am. 1973;17:651-660.

11. Kratochvil FJ. Influence of occlusal rest position and clasp design on movement of abutment teeth. J Prosthet Dent. 1963;13:114-124.

12. Krol AJ. clasp design for extension-base removable partial dentures. J Prosthet Dent. 1973;29:408-415.

13. Preston KP. The bilateral distal extension removable partial denture: mechanical problems and solutions. Eur J Prosthodont Restor Dent. 2007;15:115-121.

14. Suenaga H, Kubo K, Hosokawa R, Kuriyagawa T, Sasaki K. Effects of occlusal rest design on pressure distribution beneath the denture base of a distal extension removable partial denture-an in vivo study. Int J Prosthodont. 2014;27:469-471.

15. Zancopé K, Abrão GM, Karam FK, Neves FD. Placement of a distal implant to convert a mandibular removable Kennedy class I to an implant-supported partial removable Class III dental prosthesis: A systematic review. J Prosthet Dent. 2015;113:528-533.

Chapter 3-2.

# Combining a small number of implants to enhance RPD stability

The previous section examined how to better enhance the stability of an RPD by minimizing the force exerted on the RPD abutments. This section will focus on the ideal positioning of implants, and on how to design a small number of implants to act as abutments for an RPD. The following section will also discuss the necessity of an indirect retainer.

In this chapter, a case of a patient with a crossed occlusion will be discussed. Placing implants and designing RPDs in various intraoral situations will be examined in the next chapter.

## Question

**A female patient in her late 50s has come in for dental treatment. In this case, what would be the general treatment plan and what patient-related factors should be taken into consideration before creating an RPD?**

## Answer

The intraoral photographs taken at the time of first presentation at the clinic are shown in Figure 1.

After the consultation, the patient left to get treated at a different dental clinic and returned 2 months later with her teeth extracted as shown in Figure 2.

Patients with only unilateral residual teeth forming a crossed occlusion without any inter-occluding teeth are difficult to treat as the vertical dimension of occlusion (VDO) is unclear and the unilaterally positioned teeth make it impossible to obtain adequate stability with an RPD.

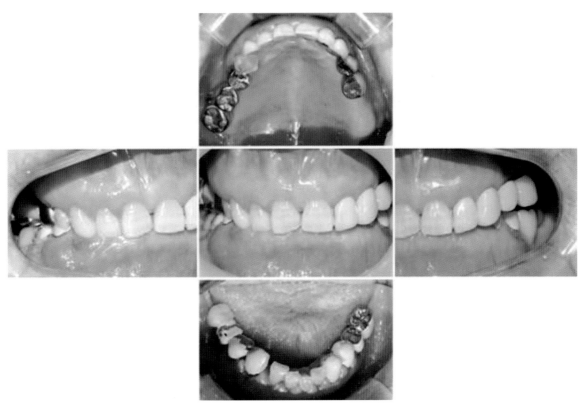

**Figure 1.** Initial intraoral photographs.

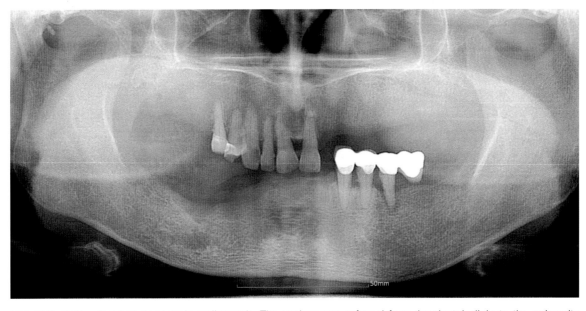

**Figure 2.** Post-extraction panoramic radiograph. The patient was referred from the dental clinic to the university dental hospital. A very typical crossed occlusion patient.

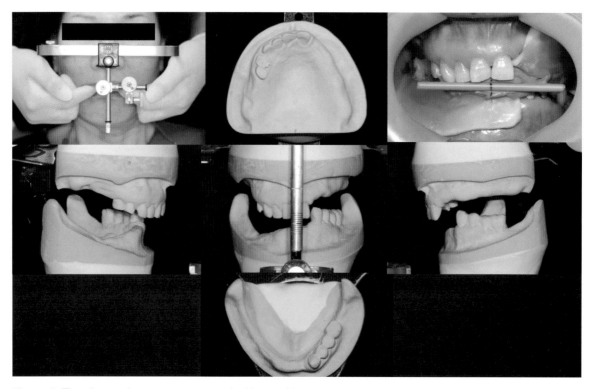

**Figure 3.** The diagnostic casts are mounted with an arbitrarily established VDO and guided centric relation.

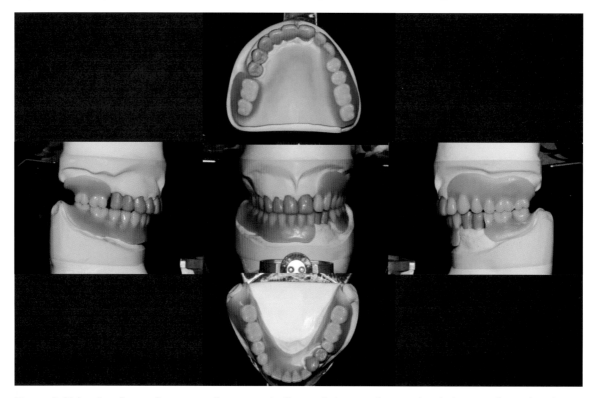

**Figure 4.** Using the diagnostic wax-up, the proper tooth morphology and an occlusal plane are formed at the arbitrarily established VDO.

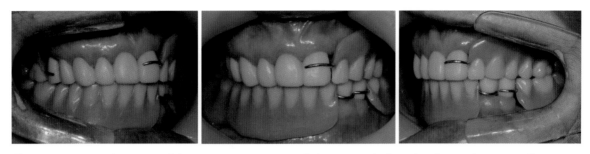

**Figure 5.** Intraoral placement of the temporary crowns and denture made from the diagnostic wax-up. Temporary prostheses are evaluated for at least 2 months to monitor the patient's adaptation to the newly formed VDO and occlusal plane. Occlusal adjustments should be made as necessary.

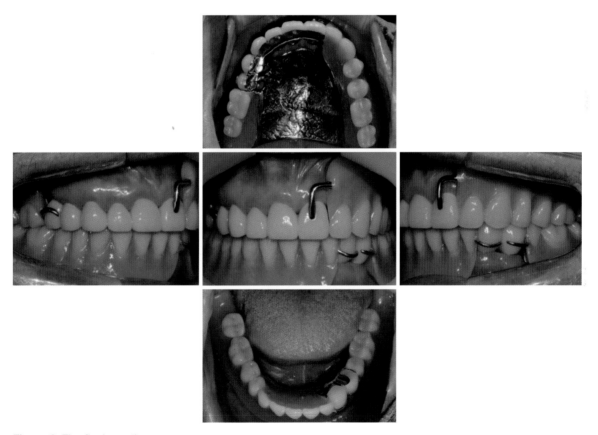

**Figure 6.** The final prostheses.

Figures 3 to 6 illustrate the stepwise approach to the treatment of this patient. The general treatment using an RPD in these kind of cases, would be to determine the proper vertical dimension of occlusion with occlusal rims to establish the proper tooth morphology and occlusal plane with diagnostic wax-ups. Based on the diagnostic wax-up, a temporary crown and denture can be fabricated. Then, these temporary

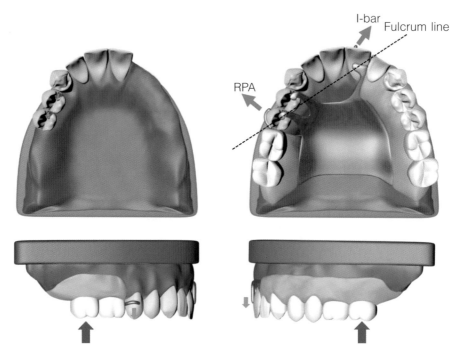

**Figure 7.** The I-bar is placed on the upper left central incisor for aesthetics. A stronger extracting force is exerted on the incisor because the I-bar is positioned anterior to the fulcrum line.

prostheses should be evaluated for 2-3 months to monitor how the patient adapts to the newly formed VDO and occlusal plane.

This case is challenging in terms of prosthodontic treatment. Not only is the fabrication of the temporary prostheses difficult, but the abutment teeth are also not stable enough for an RPD, leading to long-term complications. With the maxilla, abutment teeth are reinforced by splinting the residual teeth, and vertical support is obtained by forming a rest seat on each abutment tooth. However, the unilaterally positioned residual teeth prohibit any tissue-ward rotational freedom, even if the clasp is designed with RPI and RPA systems. In other words, unless the denture is relined regularly, it will continue to move during mastication. This means that with every mastication, the clasp positioned anterior to the fulcrum line will induce an extruding force on the abutment tooth. Furthermore, the I-bar used on the upper left central incisor for aesthetics may produce an even greater extruding force for the same reason.

With the mandible, because rests and guiding planes are only formed on the lower left canine and the first premolar, a larger amount of force is applied to the abutment teeth. Even if a wrought wire were to be used, the abutment teeth cannot last long unless sufficient stability is provided by the denture.

**What are the factors to be taken into consideration when treating patients with a crossed occlusion?**

Each patient should be given a unique, individual design that will minimize RPD movement.

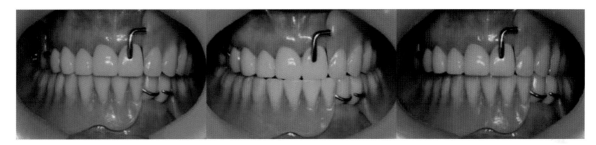

**Figure 8.** A bilaterally balanced occlusion is formed to minimize RPD movement.

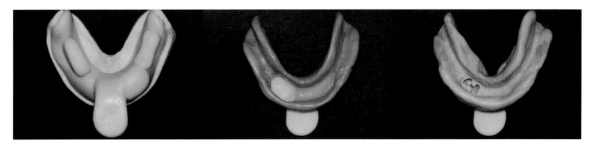

**Figure 9.** A functional impression is taken to add tissue support and RPD stability.

Dentures tend to rotate during mastication, exerting unwanted forces onto the abutment teeth. However, bilaterally balanced occlusion can reduce the rotational movement of an RPD by simultaneously forming anterior and posterior contact points during protrusion (Figure 8).

It should be noted that an impression must be carefully taken of the edentulous area for enhanced tissue support and denture stability (Figure 9). A denture reline should also be performed regularly.

**What is the ideal positioning if two implants are used as abutments for an RPD?**

In the maxilla, placing both implants on the right side is not ideal because the abutments are then positioned unilaterally. There are instead three other placement options, which are described below.

First, the two implants can be placed on the posterior region of the left maxilla, as shown in Figure 11. This is a Kennedy Class II modification 1 design. The left maxilla can now sustain a tooth-supported RPD, which is preferable when designing an RPD. However, in this case, the edentulous area between the left central incisor and the posterior implant is too wide. This may transfer an excessive force on the abutments, particularly on the left central incisor. To give a specific example, when the left mandibular canine and the first premolar are present, the possibility of the occlusal forces becoming concentrated on the edentulous area in the left maxilla cannot be overlooked. One of the problems with this design could be the location of the indirect retainer. The indirect retainer, positioned anterior to the fulcrum line, helps to maintain retention by causing the direct retainer (clasp) to fall off vertically. Here, the rest on the upper left central incisor plays the role of the indirect retainer for the distal edentulous area of the right maxilla. Though it may form an ideal rest on the incisor, a lateral force could be exerted pushing the teeth outwards. In order to prevent this, an additional splinting of the residual teeth may be needed.

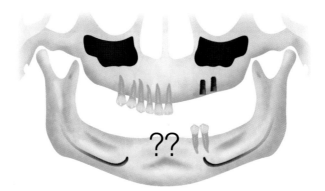

**Figure 10.** Two implants are to be placed in the maxilla as abutments for the RPD.

Second, the two implants can be placed on the upper left lateral incisor and canine, as shown in Figure 12. This treatment plan has an aesthetic advantage because of the existing incisors. However, this is considered a Kennedy Class I IARPD which may require the additional support of a fully covered

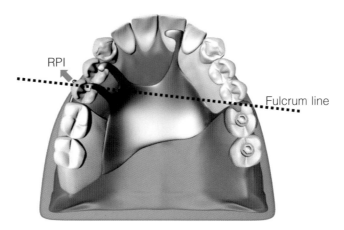

**Figure 11.** Two implants located on the maxillary left molar area.

major connector, a functional impression of the edentulous area, and occlusal consideration. Another issue may be the inability of the RPI clasp to reduce a pulling force on the abutment because of the anterior positioning of the I-bar in relation to the fulcrum line (refer to Chapter 3.1).

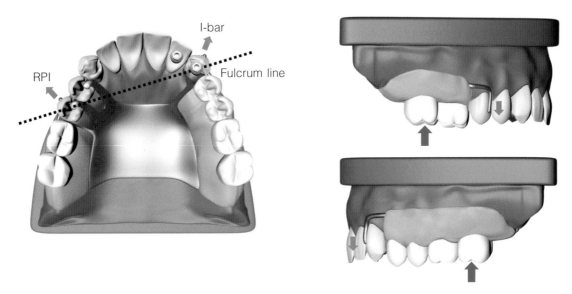

**Figure 12.** The problem with placing implants on the upper left lateral incisor and canine.

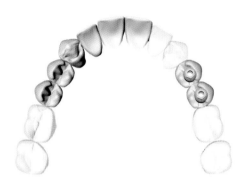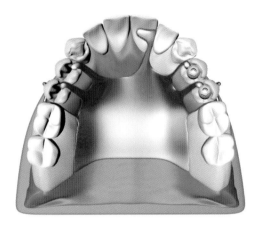

**Figure 13.** Two implants placed on the upper left first and second premolars.

Third, the two implants can be placed on the upper left first and second premolars, as shown in Figure 13. This RPD design has many advantages, one of which is that it creates bilateral symmetry in relation to the posterior abutments. With such symmetry, the clasp allows for tissue-ward movements by the denture when rotating around the fulcrum line, as previously mentioned. The vertical force on the residual teeth can be reduced by minimizing the edentulous area, and the external force can also be minimized by distributing the vertical force onto the residual ridge.

This design also ensures that the force is evenly distributed when the implants come in contact with the natural teeth, such as the lower left canine and the first premolar. When implants are placed as shown in Figure 14, the IARPD can be designed to enhance stability and to minimize the external force exerted on the abutments with additional guiding planes, the mesial rests on the implant abutments of the RPD, and symmetrically positioned abutments. It should be noted that the impression for the posterior edentulous area should be taken carefully to maintain sufficient tissue support.

In the mandible, implants can be placed on the lower right first and second premolar or canine and first premolar for a similar reason as with the maxilla. As shown in Figure 15, by placing the implants symmetrically, the fulcrum line is translocated, and the clasp allows for a tissue-ward movement of the denture base. The terminal rests on each side of the anterior edentulous area offer vertical support and act as the indirect retainer. Moreover, the occlusal force would be evenly distributed as the implants come in contact with the natural teeth.

In short, the stability of an RPD with a small number of abutments has to be established with careful

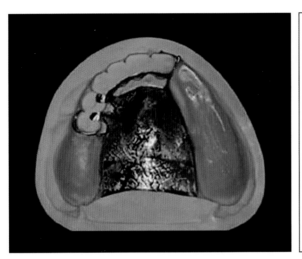 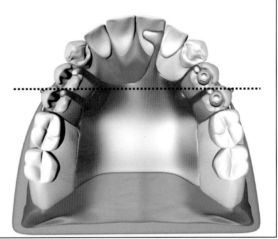

**Figure 14.** A posteriorly translocated fulcrum line enables the clasps to allow for tissue-ward movements of the denture base.

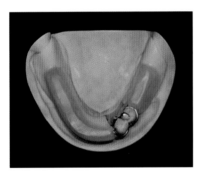 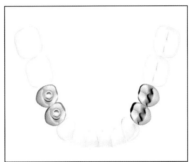 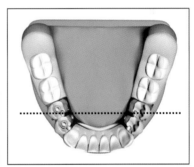

**Figure 15.** A symmetrical RPD design with implants placed on the right mandible. Rests on second premolars can be located on distal area to get wide supporting area from teeth and implants.

impression-taking on edentulous areas, regular denture relining, and occlusal adjustment. There is no single correct manual for treating patients, and appropriate treatment should be prescribed based on the aforementioned fundamental principles.

> **Keypoint**
>
> In patients with a crossed occlusion, if a small number of implants are to be used as abutments for the RPD, a symmetrical placement of the implants is recommended. In doing so, the fulcrum line can be translocated, and the indirect retainer and clasps that allow for tissue-ward movements can be properly located. Careful impressions of the supporting tissue should be taken before determining the occlusion type, and the denture stability by occlusion should be considered thereafter.

## REFERENCES

1. Avant WE. Fulcrum and retention lines in planning removable partial dentures. J Prosthet Dent. 1971;25:162-166.

2. Avant WE. Indirect retention in partial denture design. J Prosthet Dent. 1966;16:1103-1110.

3. Steffel VL. Current concepts in removable partial denture service. J Prosthet Dent. 1968;20:387-395.

*Chapter 3-3.*

# Appropriate impression-taking to enhance stability in distal extension RPDs

Chapters 3.1 and 3.2 explained how to design IARPD metal framework with enhanced stability. The importance of careful impression-taking in distal extension RPDs will be discussed in this chapter. A proper impression is necessary if the metal framework design of the RPD itself cannot prevent movement or if the use of implants or abutments is ineffective in producing sufficient stability. As previously mentioned, teeth and implants provide stability, retention, and support, so they should be evenly distributed. However, if this is insufficient, proper impressions can compensate where the teeth and/or implants fall short.

**Question**

**Is the methodology for taking impressions for an RPD the same as that for a complete denture (CD)?**

**Answer**

The methods for taking impressions in both RPDs and CDs are similar. However, it is important that the soft tissue be undisturbed while taking impressions for an RPD. As shown in Figure 1, the CD impression should cover as large an area as functionally possible to maximize retention, support, and stability throughout the denture. On the other hand, with an RPD impression, excessive coverage of soft tissue reduces its stability. In other words, the area covered by the RPD impression should not be extended excessively; the direct retainer will prevent its dislodgement. If the impression for an RPD is extended excessively, the denture will be raised repeatedly by the soft tissue during yawning or talking. Therefore, the RPD impression should cover as wide an area as possible within the limits of the tissue's

Complete denture

Removable partial denture

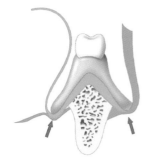

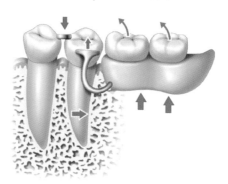

**Figure 1.** Difference between RPD and CD impressions. The RPD impression should cover as wide an area as possible within the limits of the tissue's functional movement.

functional movement, particularly because the direct retainer can extrude the abutment.

However, with this being said, it is important that the impression area is not too small. As shown in Figure 2, the denture base should at least cover the retromolar pad, press against the buccal shelf area, and extend lingually within the functional movement limitations of the tongue. The buccal shelf area provides support, and the retromolar pad and lingual extension of the denture offers stability. Generally speaking, if the patient complains of soft tissue pain with his or her RPD, the internal surface of the denture should be adjusted using a fit checker or pressure indicating paste (PIP) rather than simply reducing the length of the base of the denture. Precautions can also be taken to prevent the creation of an excessively extended base by moving the soft tissue around thoroughly during the border molding step prior to impression-taking.

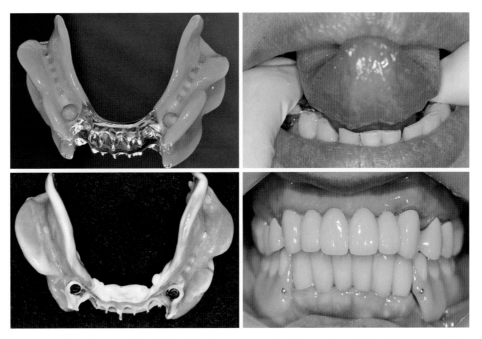

**Figure 2.** Formation of the base of the RPD following appropriate impression-taking. Coverage of the retromolar pad and lingual extension is necessary and the buccal shelf should be in full contact. Press against the occlusal rest or major connector firmly, and create movement of the soft tissue (cheek and tongue) while creating the border molding. Take precautions not to press the distal extension edentulous area during border molding, final impression-taking, and even while making adjustments on the internal surface of the denture.

> **Keypoint**
>
> Press against the occlusal rest firmly to generate cheek and tongue movement while border molding of the denture. Ensure that when the denture is seated completely, the movement of soft tissue (cheek or tongue) is not interrupted. In an RPD, only the occlusal rest or major connectors should be pressed; the distal extension edentulous area of the RPD should be left unpressed during all processes, including impression-taking, adjustment making, and relining.

**Question**

**What parts of the maxilla and mandible should be covered for a distal extension RPD?**

**Answer**

In the maxilla, the parts indicated in yellow in Figure 3 below should be left untouched. The crestal ridge, responsible for vertical support, is called the 'primary stress-bearing area'. This area is comprised of firm fibrous connective tissues covering the cortical bone, which explains why this area can resist vertical

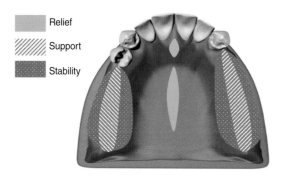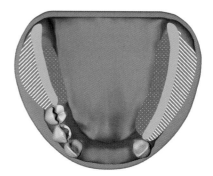

| | |
|---|---|
| Relief | |
| Support | |
| Stability | |

**Figure 3.** Roles of various edentulous parts in maxilla and mandible.

forces effectively. The area colored with dotted lines provides stability. As the slope becomes steeper and longer, stability is enhanced, particularly in the maxilla.

Impression-taking is particularly difficult with distal extension areas in the mandible (Figure 3). Unlike in the maxilla, the crestal ridge and retromolar pad should not be pressed in the mandible. If firm connective tissue is present on the retromolar pad, it can be pressed. However, in general, the retromolar pad is mostly covered by thick, mobile soft tissue. The region marked with stripes indicates the buccal shelf, which mainly offers support, but also enhances the stability. The area colored in orange indicates the lingual denture base area, which mainly offers additional stability. Extending this area sufficiently can also prevent the horizontal rotation of RPD.

### Question

**Many patients experience discomfort with a distal extension RPD in the mandible. How can enhanced support and stability in the mandible be achieved during impression-taking?**

### Answer

Figure 4A shows that with a tooth-supported RPD, the support provided by the soft tissue is not necessarily important because the tooth itself offers vertical support. With a distal extension RPD (Figure 4B), however, tissue support is extremely important because the RPD may undergo a tissue-ward movement. In order to enhance support, functional and selective pressure impressions can be taken. The

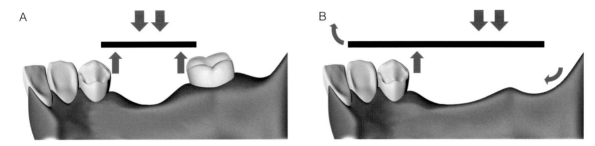

**Figure 4.** Difference in support offered by tooth-supported and tooth- and tissue-supported RPDs.

remaining teeth can provide sufficient support and stability in a distal extension RPD; enhancing support with the denture itself is not of utmost importance.

As previously mentioned, taking the impression for the mandible of a distal extension RPD is difficult because generating the appropriate amount of pressure to support the buccal shelf area is challenging.

Figure 5 shows the cross-sectional view of the mandible. The buccal shelf region is covered with thick and elastic soft tissue. In contrast, the crestal ridge and lingual areas are covered with a thinner layer of soft tissue. As such, a larger amount of pressure can be exerted on the thick soft tissue on the buccal shelf area, and because of its elasticity, the tissue will quickly recover to its buoyant state following denture removal.

The buccal shelf area is the first part that will receive pressure upon insertion of the RPD. Following an occlusion, the force is first distributed to the soft tissue of the buccal shelf area, and contact with points B, C, and D as shown in Figure 5 occurs simultaneously and uniformly thereafter.

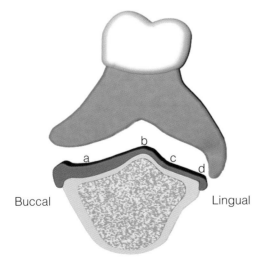

Buccal

Lingual

**Figure 5.** Cross sectional view of the mandible. Buccal shelf area is covered with thick and firm soft tissue, and the crestal and lingual area is covered with thin soft tissue.

Figure 6A displays how an RPD would be inserted without an occlusion; the buccal shelf area will be in contact, but the denture will remain suspended above the other areas. With the occlusal force, however, the pressure distribution is similar to what is shown in Figure 6B. Creating an impression similar to the one displayed as in Figure 6 requires the use of more pressure than an anatomical impression. The denture base should be shaped so that it presses perfectly against the soft tissue. This impression-taking method is called the 'selective pressure impression method', and yields favorable results.

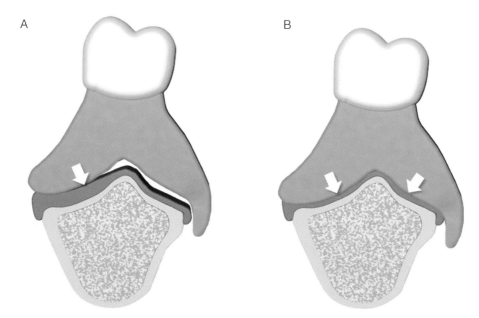

**Figure 6.** Denture base pressing against the soft tissue with occlusal force. (A) Pressure is exerted upon the buccal shelf area first during the insertion of an RPD. (B) When RPD is seated fully with occlusal force, every soft tissue is contacted with denture base.

### Question

**Given that a functional impression can provide support for a distal extension RPD, in what ways does it also enhance stability?**

### Answer

A tissue-ward movement about the most posterior abutment tooth can be prevented with a functional impression because it offers enhanced support in the distal edentulous region (Figure 7).

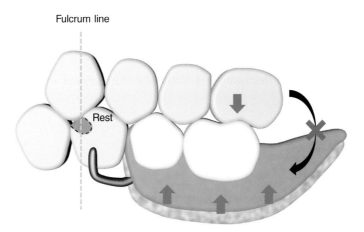

**Figure 7.** Increased support in the buccal shelf area prevents tissue-ward movements of the denture.

Besides, a rotational movement around the longitudinal axis formed by the crest of the residual ridge (often leading to the lifting of the denture) can also be prevented.

The Pound's line should be used as a reference point when arranging artificial teeth on the distal edentulous areas for a distal extension RPD of mandible. The Pound's line connects the mesial contact point of the canine to the buccal and lingual border of the retromolar pad. Lingual cusps of the mandibular posterior teeth should be placed in the triangular region formed by Pound's line. Even if there is substantial buccal bone resorption, the artificial teeth should still be placed in the same position. In this case, the buccal cusp, the functional cusp of the mandible, will be placed more on the buccal side than on the

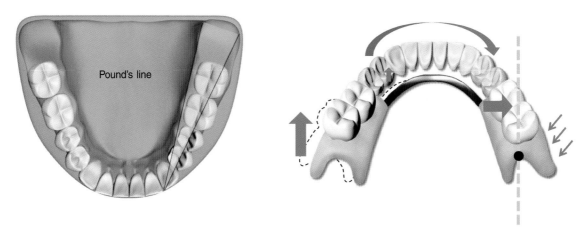

**Figure 8.** A rotational movement around the longitudinal axis formed by the crest of the residual ridge can be prevented.

crest of the residual ridge. This creates a Class I lever when an occlusal force is applied, with the crest acting as the fulcrum. If the denture is created with a well-made buccal shelf impression, it will then firmly press against the buccal shelf, decreasing the likelihood of rotational movement. This ensures the patient's comfort during mastication.

**How much pressure can be exerted while taking an impression of the buccal shelf area?**

The process of taking a selective pressure impression can be applied here.

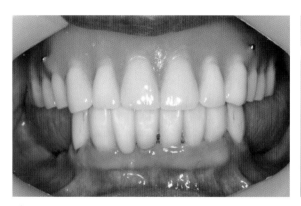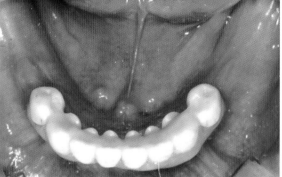

**Figure 9.** Patient with a bilateral distal edentulous area in the mandible. Severe alveolar bone resorption of the edentulous area in the mandible. Abutment teeth extend up to both first premolars with splinting, and lingual rests are properly formed in all teeth.

As shown in Figure 11, after utilizing the fit checker on the metal framework, press firmly on it without pressing against the distal edentulous areas. A selective pressure impression should offer vertical support to the abutment during mastication, and the vertical force applied must be distributed evenly to the soft tissue on the edentulous areas. Therefore, when adjusting the metal framework, special care should be taken to ensure that it fits appropriately. Adjustments should continue to be made until the metal framework is perfectly fitted and the rest is fully seated. An ill-fitting RPD may transfer excessive force to the abutment teeth and the lateral rotational force may also be transferred to the implants.

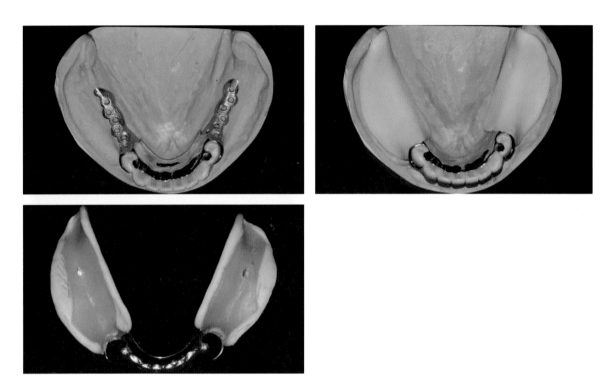

**Figure 10.** A resin tray is created on the metal framework placed on the edentulous areas. For border molding, form a tray border about 0.5~1.0 mm shorter than the border shown in the model. The tray is fabricated with a sheet of base plate wax on the edentulous area for impression material space.

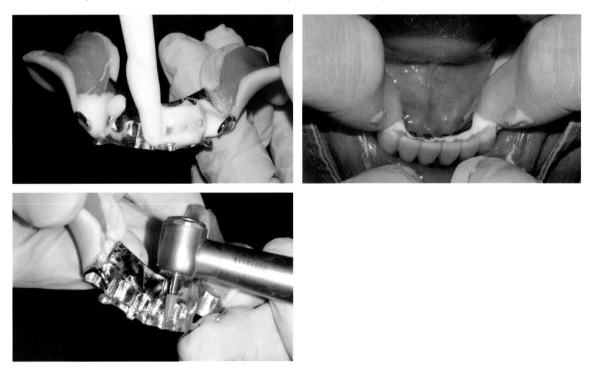

**Figure 11.** Internal fit test of the metal framework. If the metal framework does not sit properly, a functional impression cannot be accurately taken.

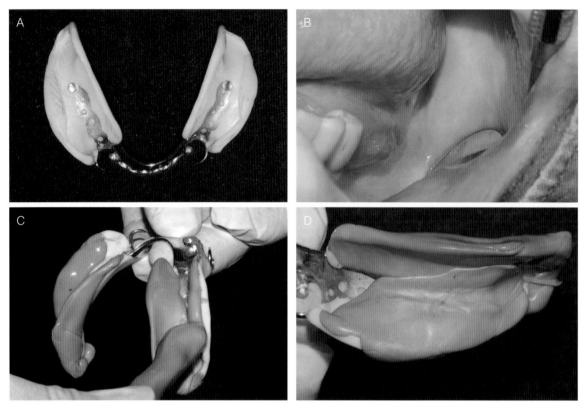

**Figure 12.** Border molding process using a modeling compound. One-step border molding materials such as silicone can be used for functional impressions.

Removal of the internal wax and replacement by the modeling compound are important steps in border molding (Figure 12). Patients with severe bone resorption may appear to have a small buccal shelf area, but if the cheek is stretched apart, the entire buccal shelf area becomes exposed. It is important to take the impression all the way until the external oblique ridge is covered. The modeling compound can capture the entire length of the border as well as the status of the internal surface of the soft tissue. It is important that the border molding process be done by pressing only the rests (and major connector).

It is imperative that pressure is exerted only upon the appropriate areas during impression-taking. The modeling compound can be checked to see if pressure was placed on the wrong areas, as there will be additional indentations in the impression. Adjustments can be made after the altered cast is made or during the final RPD delivery and try-in.

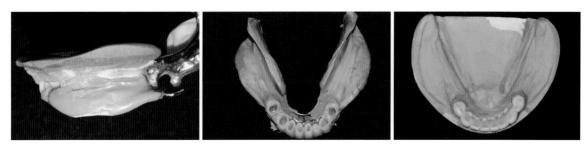

**Figure 13.** After molding the border, reduce the border length and internal surface of the modeling compound without touching the buccal shelf area.

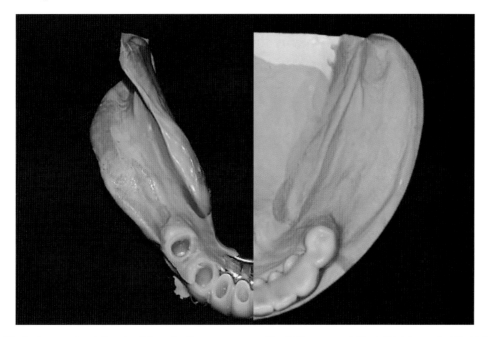

**Figure 14.** An impression taken by this selective pressure methodology can capture the intraoral state in its entirety, ranging from the residual ridge to the altered cast. If the selective pressure impression is taken properly, the buccal shelf area should be seen, as shown in the figure on the left.

---

**Keypoint**

Only the occlusal rest (or major connector) should be pressed when taking the impression with a modeling compound. A modeling compound that is not fully softened may require excessive pressure, it is therefore important to ensure that the compound has been fully softened.

---

When a selective pressure impression is taken correctly, a greater amount of the soft tissue can be pressed, and this yields a better impression of the buccal shelf area. The resulting denture is larger but can be easily adjusted post-fabrication. If the new RPD results in soreness or pain on the lingual surface, it means that the buccal shelf region lacks support. In this case, adding on to the buccal shelf area may be the solution, but this is far more challenging than grinding down an excessively large denture.

### Question

**Situation 1.** **Post-RPD delivery, a patient comes in with ulcers and redness on areas of soft tissue in contact with the lingual flange of the denture.**

**Situation 2.** **Post-RPD delivery, a patient complains of pain resulting from the buccal shelf being uncomfortably pressed by the denture.**

**Which situation is better to control?**

### Answer

Situation 1 occurs when the buccal shelf offers insufficient support and the internal surface of the denture ends up pressing against the lingual soft tissue. Unfortunately, this requires that new impressions or reline be taken, this time with more pressure exerted on the buccal shelf area.

Situation 2 occurs when the buccal shelf area is pressed with too much force during impression-taking. In this case, selectively grinding off parts of the denture, particularly on the buccal shelf area, is necessary.

Generally, adding on to the internal surface of the denture base is more difficult than grinding the internal surface of the denture base.

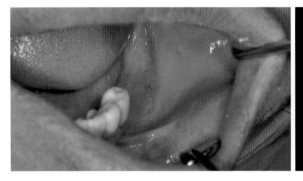 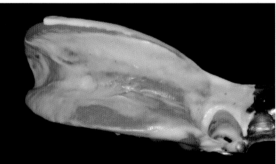

**Figure 15.** When excessive pressure is exerted on the buccal shelf area while taking the impression, the patient may experience redness and ulcerations. However, this type of denture is easier to adjust, given that an entirely new set of impressions does not have to be taken.

### Question

## Should impressions be taken with selective pressure for all distal extension RPDs?

### Answer

Selective pressure impressions should be taken when insufficient teeth are remaining, and when more than three teeth on both molar regions are missing in a Kennedy Class I patient, and when more than 3 teeth on molar regions on the mandible are missing in a Kennedy Class II patient. In tooth-supported RPDs, an anatomical impression can be taken, and in other cases requiring a distal extension RPD, both an anatomical impression of the teeth and a selective pressure impression of the soft tissue can be taken simultaneously by a one-step method using a single tray. Figure 16 is an author's flowchart indicating how to determine what type of impression should be taken.

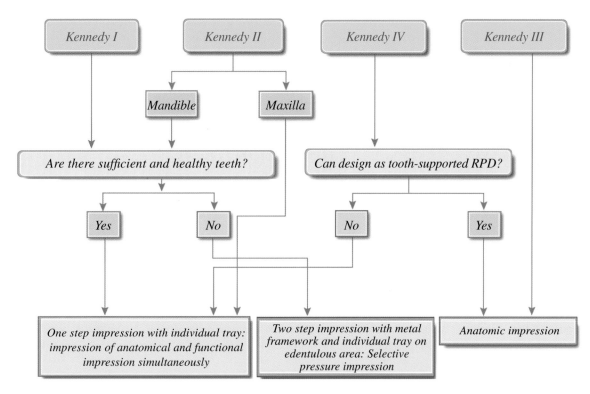

**Figure 16.** A flowchart indicating how to determine what type of impression should be taken.

**Question**

**What is a one-step impression using an individual tray, and how does it differ from a two-step impression?**

**Answer**

In a selective pressure impression, two steps are needed in that the metal framework is first created, and then the impressions of the distal extension areas are taken. One-step impression, introduced by Herman et al.(1998), involves taking impressions of the abutment teeth and the edentulous areas simultaneously on the same tray.

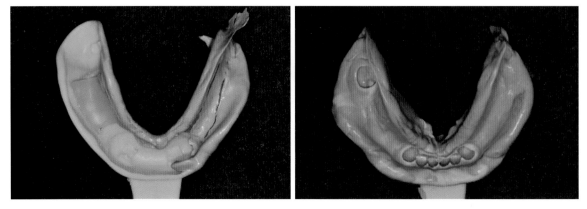

**Figure 17.** Semi-functional impression (selective pressure single impression procedure). Anatomical impression of the remaining teeth and selective pressure impression of the edentulous area are taken simultaneously with one tray.

The purpose of taking a selective pressure impression after creating the metal framework is to use the framework as a reference point to position the tray for the impression. This ensures that the tray of the edentulous area can be positioned accurately. However, a semi-functional impression (selective pressure single impression procedure) can take both the anatomical impression of the abutment teeth and the

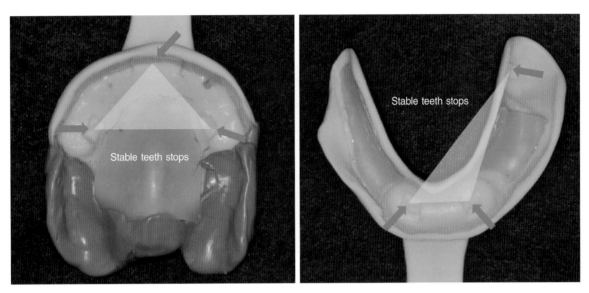

**Figure 18.** Making a stable tray without any movement by using stops on the abutment teeth area.

functional impression of the edentulous regions simultaneously, though with an ambiguous reference point.

Similar to how the metal framework can act as a reference point, 2-3 stops can be positioned onto a tray to ensure its stability during semi-functional impression-taking.

As shown in Figure 18, the tray can be positioned appropriately without any movement when it has three stable positioning stops. In this case, the edentulous areas should not be pressed during impression-taking. Remember to take a selective pressure impression of the distal edentulous area without any movement of the tray by pressing firmly on the stops of the abutment teeth area.

> **Keypoint**
>
> Placing stable positioning stops is of utmost importance for a one-step impression to guarantee tray stability. Similar to the two-step impression utilizing a metal framework, if there are not enough teeth present to apply stable positioning stops on the tray, the impression should be taken as if it were being taken for a complete denture.

# REFERENCES

1. Chen MS, Eichhold WA, Chien CC, Curtis DA. An altered-cast impression technique that eliminates conventional cast dissecting and impression boxing. J Prosthet Dent. 1987;57:471-474.

2. Herman B. Selective pressure single impression procedure for tooth-mucosa-support removable partial dentures. J Prosthet Dent. 1998;80:259-261.

3. Jacobson TE, Krol AJ. A contemporary review of the factors involved in complete dentures. Part III: support. J Prosthet Dent. 1983;49:306-313.

4. Leupold RJ, Flinton RJ, Pfeifer DL. Comparison of vertical movement occurring during loading of distal-extension removable partial denture bases made by three impression techniques. J Prosthet Dent. 1992;68:290-293.

5. Leupold RJ, Kratochvil FJ. An altered-cast procedure to improve tissue support for removable partial dentures. J Prosthet Dent. 1965;15:672-678.

6. Lund PS, Aquilino SA. Prefabricated custom impression trays for the altered cast technique. J Prosthet Dent. 1991;66:782-783.

7. McCarthy JA, Moser JB. Tissue conditioning and functional impression materials and techniques. Dental Clinics of North America. 1984;28:239.

8. Monteith BD. Management of loading forces on mandibular distal-extension prostheses. Part I: Evaluation of concepts for design. J Prosthet Dent. 1984;52:673-681.

9. Monteith BD. Management of loading forces on mandibular distal-extension prostheses. Part II: Classification for matching modalities to clinical situations. J Prosthet Dent. 1984;52:832-836.

Chapter 3-4.

# Understanding how an occlusion can enhance the stability of the RPD

Minimizing the lateral rotational force exerted on the implant by enhancing the stability of the RPD is of the utmost importance when treating a patient with an IARPD. It has been previously established that adjustments can be made to the metal framework to create a more stable RPD. However, if the support provided by this is still insufficient, creating a perfectly harmonized occlusion is the next step to manufacturing a stable RPD.

It is imperative that the patient's occlusal scheme is left undisturbed if it is already well-balanced. In attempting to achieve well-balanced and harmonized oral movements in edentulous patients, dentists may make adjustments to occlusal factors, but should never change the patient's condylar guidance. As such, in partially edentulous patients, dentists should first check whether the residual teeth form a well-balanced and harmonious occlusion, and only make adjustments if necessary. Also, the occlusal surface of the artificial teeth should be similar in shape to that of the residual natural teeth.

### Question

**How can a stable occlusion be formed with an IARPD?**

### Answer

Achieving occlusal stability in an IARPD is not too different from how it is achieved in a conventional RPD. However, extra care should be taken when making occlusal adjustments in patients with an IARPD, which uses natural teeth abutments. Some suggestions towards extra care are listed below:

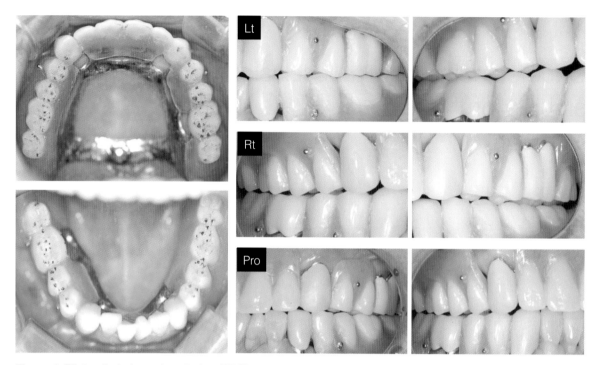

**Figure 1.** Bilaterally balanced occlusion (BBO) and precise occlusal contact of molars in centric relation (CR) or maximum intercuspal position (MICP).

(1) The molars should come in contact bilaterally and evenly in centric occlusion or maximum intercuspal position (MICP). Particularly with IARPDs, there must be sufficient support provided by the molars when they come in contact.

(2) A bilaterally balanced occlusion (BBO) should be formed during eccentric movements when the mandibular RPD occludes with the maxillary complete denture (Figure 2).

Additionally, as shown in Figure 3, if the patient has a large edentulous area, indicative of frequent movement of the RPD, creating a BBO is of even greater importance.

Generally, a BBO will contribute to the stability of maxillary complete dentures during lateral movements. However, when the incisors and molars occlude simultaneously during protrusive movements, creating occlusal plane disharmony, aesthetics and pronunciation should take priority over a balanced occlusion.

(3) Furthermore, a BBO should also be considered for Kennedy Class I RPD cases.

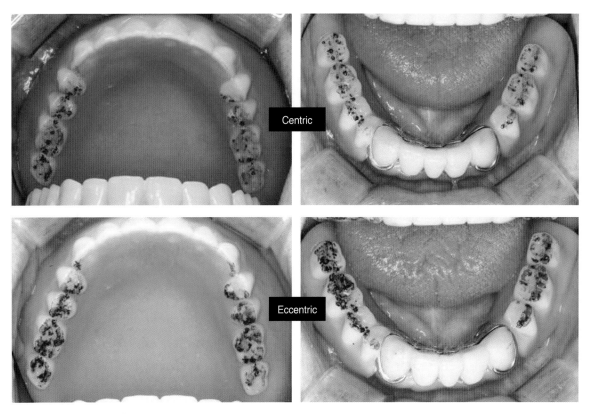

**Figure 2.** The patient is expected to experience frequent movement with an IARPD due to a large edentulous area. A BBO can still be successfully formed with the upper complete denture occluding with a lower IARPD.

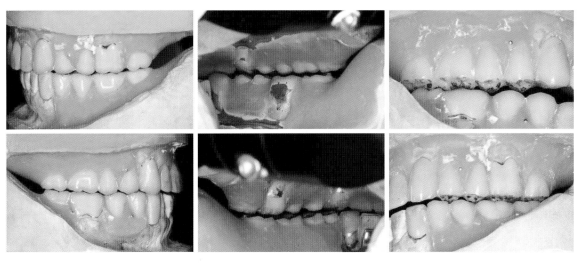

**Figure 3.** In patients with a mandibular bilateral distal extension RPD and an insufficient number of abutment teeth (especially in an IARPD), a bilaterally balanced occlusion can reduce the excessive lateral rotational movement of the RPD.

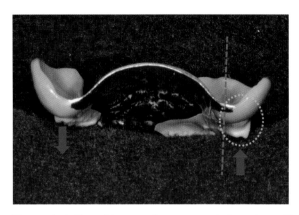 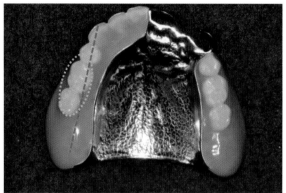

**Figure 4.** A Class I lever action may result from the artificial teeth being arranged in the buccal part of the crestal ridge (due to severe bone resorption). In such cases, extra stability can be provided with a proper occlusion.

As shown in Figure 4, extensive buccal resorption of the alveolar bone in the maxillary is common in long-term edentulous patients. In most of these cases, the artificial teeth in the maxillary RPDs are arranged on the buccal part of the alveolar ridge, and rotational movement occurs about the longitudinal axis formed by the crest of the residual ridge during mastication. Therefore, in such cases, a BBO should be formed under the consideration that the denture base has a good adaptation with the soft tissue area. The concept of forming a BBO should not be limited to the case in which the opposing dentition is a complete denture, and an appropriate occlusal relation should be formed based on the biomechanics around the rotational axis. In this case, an additional implant can be placed to prevent the RPD's unwanted movements. The intentional crossbite occlusion in posterior artificial teeth may also prevent the rotational movement of the RPD, but the patient may experience some discomfort because of the crossbite arrangement of the artificial teeth.

However, it should be noted that if the patient has a deep bite (slight horizontal overjet or excessive overbite), reduction and re-restoration of the anterior teeth may be necessary. Keep in mind that if the patient does not experience any discomfort with his or her existing occlusion, unnecessary adjustments should not be made. If the residual teeth are healthy or if more than two stable implants have been installed and splinted, the movement of an RPD should be limited with canine guidance, group function, a unilaterally balanced occlusion, or a crossbite instead.

**Question**

**What can be done to create a proper occlusion when the RPD lacks stability?**

**Answer**

The following steps should be followed to establish a proper occlusion with an IARPD that experiences excessive movement.

(1) Once the metal framework is fabricated, any unnecessary contact points formed should be removed to enable smooth insertion of the metal framework. However, the contact areas formed by the clasp

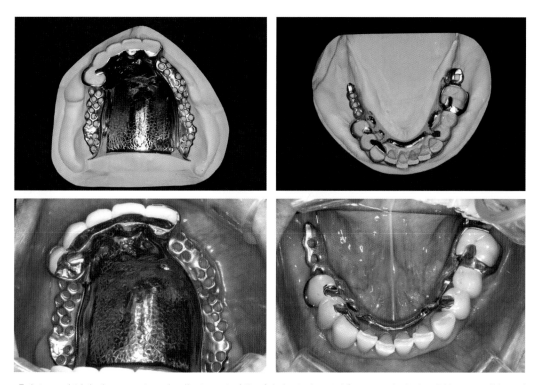

**Figure 5.** Intraoral trial-placement and adjustment of the fabricated metal framework. It should be possible to insert the metal framework passively and all the rests should be perfectly seated.

assembly should remain intact, as it provides the necessary retention and stability (reciprocation), as shown in Figure 5.

(2) Forming a resin recording base with an occlusal rim made with baseplate wax on a metal framework and obtaining a precise bite registration are fundamental steps in forming a proper occlusion. Obtaining a bite registration made only from wax on a metal framework must be avoided because the wax can be distorted, resulting in an inaccurate bite registration (Figure 6).

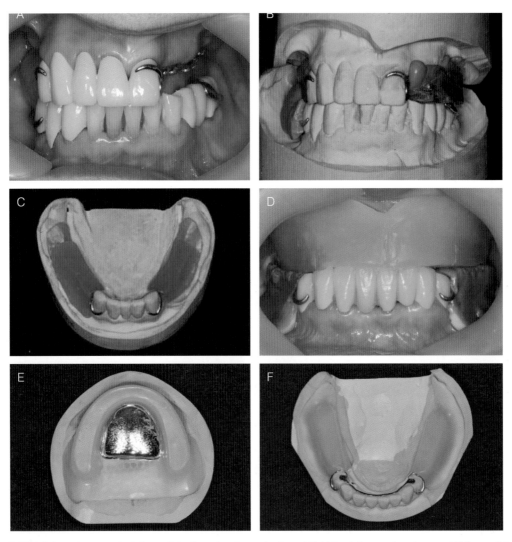

**Figure 6.** Obtaining an accurate bite registration. As shown in A and B, if the inter-occlusal record (bite registration) is taken on a base made from silicone, the inter-occlusal record may be distorted due to the silicone's elasticity. Similarly, if the record base is made with wax, as shown in C (lower jaw) and D (upper jaw), the impression may also become distorted. Therefore, it is best to take an inter-occlusal record on an occlusal rim built on a metal framework, or on a resin recording base, as shown in E and F.

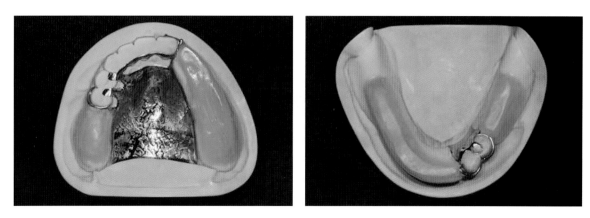

**Figure 7.** The recording base should be formed from acrylic resin to get an accurate bite registration.

(3) After arranging the maxillary and mandibular posterior teeth and receiving the wax trial dentures, the dentist should perform occlusal adjustments. If the wax dentures result in an improper occlusion, then inter-occlusal records should be taken again and the casts should be remounted. If a BBO needs to be formed, the dentist should ask for a uniform occlusal contact on the working side,

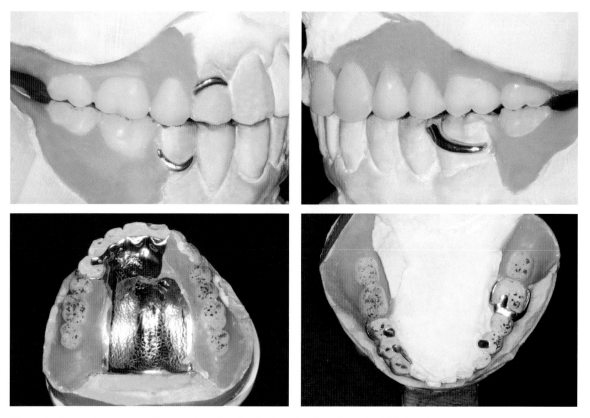

**Figure 8.** Laboratory remounting and occlusal adjustments done in a dental laboratory.

and at least 2 or 3 contact points on the non-working side. Producing an RPD with a BBO that has every tooth in contact on the non-working side (balancing side) is very challenging. Adequate stability can be achieved with just two occlusal contact points on the non-working side.

(4) As shown in Figure 8, after curing the wax denture, laboratory remounting is necessary to adjust the errors made during the resin curing process. These adjustments are typically made in a dental laboratory, but it is advisable for the dentist to polish the dentures themselves after checking whether the desired occlusion has been formed. This stage requires full cooperation between the dentist and dental technician, as further intraoral adjustments are difficult after this step.

(5) If proper occlusal adjustments are made during the laboratory remounting process, further occlusal adjustments through clinical remounting are not necessary. However, if there are still excessive errors to be fixed, clinical remounting may be necessary. As shown in Figure 9, additional occlusal adjustments can be made after the clinical remounting process.

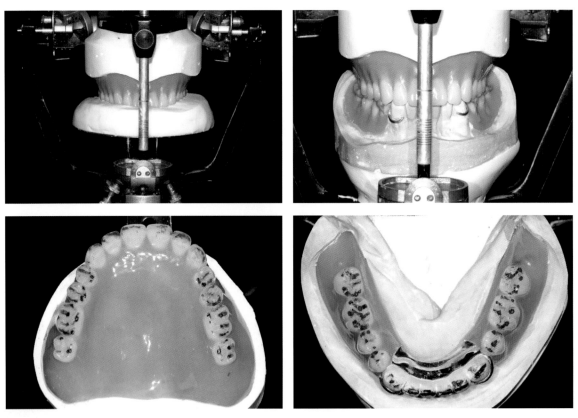

**Figure 9.** Clinical remounting. If the IARPD is ill-fitting and needs to be adjusted intraorally, the dentist can make further adjustments after clinical remounting.

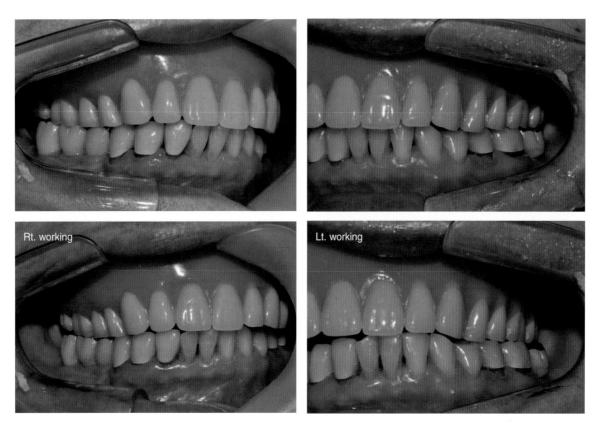

**Figure 10.** Intraoral examination being completed after clinical remounting. A proper BBO can be obtained.

The use of implants requires extra care at each step of the treatment process. Attempting to enhance stability by adjusting the occlusion should only be resorted to when all other steps have been taken, including designing a supportive metal framework as well as taking proper impressions.

# REFERENCES

1. Hämmerle CH, Wagner D, Bragger U, Lussi A, Karayiannis A, Joss A, Lang NP. Threshold of tactile sensitivity perceived with dental endosseous implants and natural teeth. Clin Oral Implants Res. 1995;6:83–90.

2. Isidor F. Loss of osseointegration caused by occlusal load of oral implants. A clinical and radiographic study in monkeys. Clin Oral Implants Res. 1996;7:143–152.

3. Kim Y, Oh TJ, Misch CE, Wang H. Occlusal considerations in implant therapy: clinical guidelines with biomechanical rationale. Clin Oral Implants Res. 2005;16:26-35.

4. Peroz I, Leuenberg A, Haustein I, Lange KP. Comparison between balanced occlusion and canine guidance in complete denture wearers – a clinical, randomized trial. Quintessence Int. 2003;34:607–612.

5. Wismeijer D, van Waas MA, Kalk W. Factors to consider in selecting an occlusal concept for patients with implants in the edentulous mandible. J Prosthet Dent. 1995;74:380–384.

*Chapter 3-5.*

# Appropriate relining techniques can yield additional stability in the RPD

When using a small number of implants for the RPD, resorption of the alveolar bone in the tissue often causes the denture to be ill-fitting. As a result, the likelihood of an anteroposterior rotation about the most posterior abutment is increased, particularly for a Kennedy Class I RPD. Therefore, proper relining of the IARPD is crucial to prevent excessive exertion of lateral and rotational forces upon the abutments.

As with complete dentures, relining RPDs can create a better fitting denture. As shown in Figure 1, the stability of occlusion and the condition of the denture determines whether the denture requires relining, rebasing, reconstruction or reproduction.

This chapter will focus mainly on relining. If a reline is performed periodically to prevent RPD movement, dentures should truly never reach the point of needing a rebase procedure.

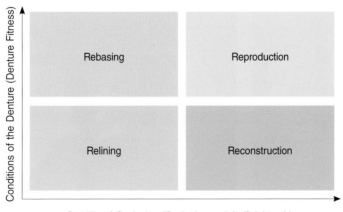

**Figure 1.** Denture repair methods depend on the stability of occlusion and the condition of the denture.

## Question

At what point is a reline of the maxilla and mandible necessary?

## Answer

In the mandibular Kennedy Class I RPD, a reline is necessary if the rests become lifted due to an anteroposterior rotation of the denture that occurs when the molar area is pushed downward (Figure 2). A fit checker can be used to determine this as well.

However, there are many other cases in which a maxillary RPD requires relining, even when the rests are not lifted upon pressure exertion. This is because the palate provides additional vertical support. Instead, the necessity of a reline can be determined by examining the level of alveolar bone resorption using a fit checker or pressure indicating paste (PIP). If the posterior edentulous area in an IARPD that uses a small number of implants or attachments is pressed down as shown in Figure 2, and the rest is clearly lifted, it is likely that excessive lateral rotational force is already being applied to the implant and natural teeth.

If a reline is necessary, the indirect relining method should be followed. First, reduce the inner-thickness of the denture base by 1 mm in all areas except for the buccal shelf. This step is similar to a selective pressure impression. If necessary, a border mold can also be made. A silicone impression can then be used to take an impression of the distal extension area. Ensure that only the rests or major connectors are pressed down while taking the impression. The resulting impression can then be sent to a dental laboratory to be replaced with acrylic resin.

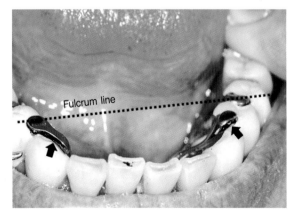
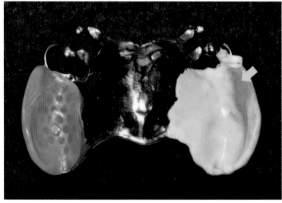

**Figure 2.** Methods to determine the necessity of a reline in maxillary and mandibular dentures.

**What are the essential points to be kept in mind for a reline?**

The indirect and direct relining methods do not differ significantly. The indirect method requires the impression of the edentulous region to be sent to a dental laboratory to be replaced by an acrylic resin, as shown in Figure 3. The direct method is a chairside reline, using autopolymerizing acrylic resin. Both methods have their merits, but the indirect method is preferred if a lot of resin needs to be added, and the direct method is preferred when the reline requires the addition of a small

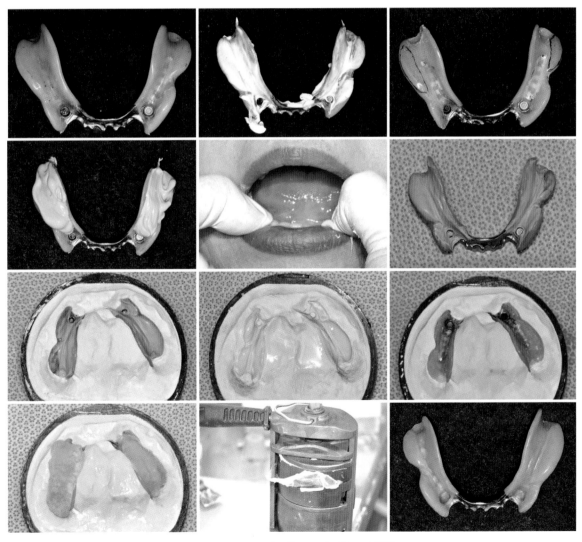

**Figure 3.** The indirect relining process in a mandibular Kennedy Class I RPD.

amount of resin. A direct reline is performed more frequently, as dentures should be checked and relined at least once a year. Indirect relines are indicative of more severe distortions present in the RPD. As such, the following sections will focus on the direct relining process.

> **Keypoint**
>
> Three important points that should be emphasized are: (1) an open-mouth technique must be used, and the patient should never bite down during the relining process; (2) the rests on abutments or major connectors must be pressed firmly, without pressing the posterior edentulous area (3) after the reline is complete, occlusal adjustments must be made.

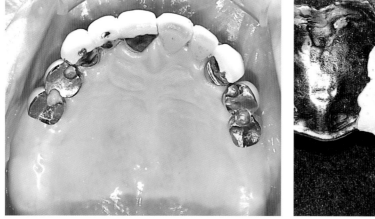 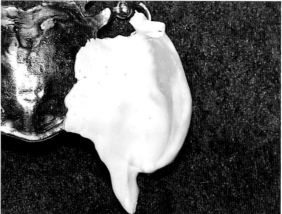

**Figure 4.** The evaluation of an IARPD with bilaterally placed implants in the premolar areas.

Figure 4 displays a case in which the bilateral implants on the first and second maxillary premolars were performed 6 years ago. The patient did not experience any discomfort during the last check-up. However, there were no stable occlusal contact points on the molars, and a slight redness was found on the buccal part of the posterior edentulous area. Accordingly, adjustments were made. As shown in Figure 4, slight alveolar bone resorption on the edentulous area was observed.

There are many cases in which patients with short edentulous areas in the maxilla do not experience any discomfort even if their dentures are in a state that requires a reline. This is because adequate support is provided by the major connectors covering the palate and teeth supported by the rests. When the molar occlusal support weakens and the denture's fit begins to falter, a relining should be performed as soon as possible. When it is not treated, patients may masticate with the anterior implant prostheses, and not with the RPD. A lateral rotational force may then be continuously transferred to the implant because of the ill-fitting denture.

Only the rests of the RPD should be pressed while conducting fit checks. The patient must not close his or her mouth. The clinician must not press the posterior edentulous areas of the RPD. This is called the open-mouth technique, which is commonly applied in selective pressure impression-taking, relining, and fit checks.

Figure 5 explains the reason why an open-mouth technique must be used in an adaptation check or relining. When the RPD is first fabricated, it has a proper inter-occlusal relationship as shown in Figure 5A. As shown in Figure 5B, following alveolar bone resorption, the posterior part of the RPD undergoes a tissue-ward rotation, and the occlusal contact points between the maxillary molars and mandibular artificial teeth are lost. The maxillary molars then will extrude as shown in Figure 5C. At this point, if a reline is performed using the closed-mouth technique, there is no point in making the adjustments and there is no meaning of reline.

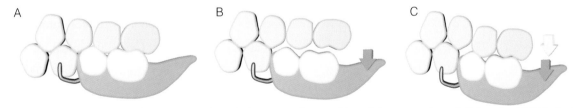

**Figure 5.** The reason why the open-mouth technique must be used in relining procedure. A: When the RPD is first fabricated, B: Following alveolar bone resorption, the posterior part of the RPD undergoes a tissue ward rotation, C: Opposing teeth are extruded.

As shown in Figure 6, use a denture bur to shave down the area needing a reline. Usually, it is recommended to file down the denture at least 1 mm to allow sufficient thickness for the reline resin. In a direct reline, the thin layer of the newly applied relined resin is often pulled apart from the existing denture base.

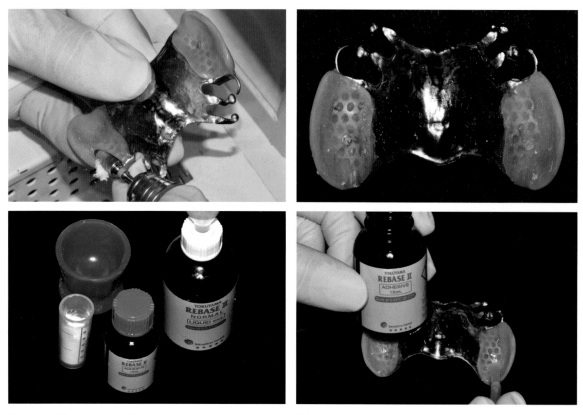

**Figure 6.** Shaving down the area needing a reline and applying adhesive or primer on the inner surface of denture base. It is recommended to file down the denture at least 1 mm to allow sufficient thickness for the reline resin.

The most challenging part of doing a direct reline is ensuring the exclusion of any bubbles. Therefore, the mixing process is particularly important. Unfortunately, there is no definite solution to this issue. However, certain precautions can be taken to minimize the number of air bubbles formed during the mixing process. Figure 7A shows the initial state of the materials to be mixed. Often, the initial mixture is very thin and watery. After 30 to 60 seconds, however, it becomes more viscous, as shown in Figure 7B. Once it reaches this stage, it can be applied to the denture. Excessive and unnecessary mixing is never recommended. After gentle mixing, some air bubbles may be present, as shown in Figure 7C. Gently tap the rubber cup against a flat surface after gently mixing to let the air bubbles escape. The remaining bubbles can be removed with a spatula from the surface of the mixture. As shown in Figure 7D, after removing all the large bubbles from the surface, apply the resin onto the denture. Figures 7E and F were taken under an optical microscope. Figure 7E shows the state of the mixture in 7C, and Figure 7F shows the state of the mixture in 7D after bubbles have been removed.

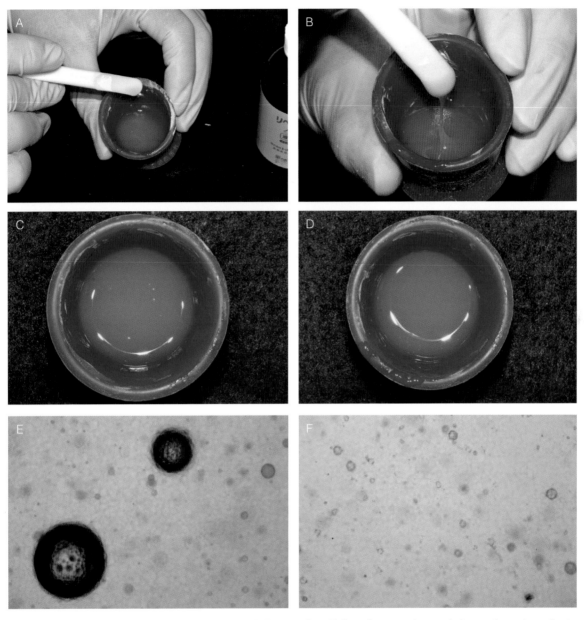

**Figure 7.** Mixing and applying the acrylic resin during a reline. Follow the manufacturer's instructions. In order to reduce the number of bubbles in the resin, mix slowly, taking great care. E shows the state of the mixture in C, and F shows the state of the mixture in D after bubbles have been removed.

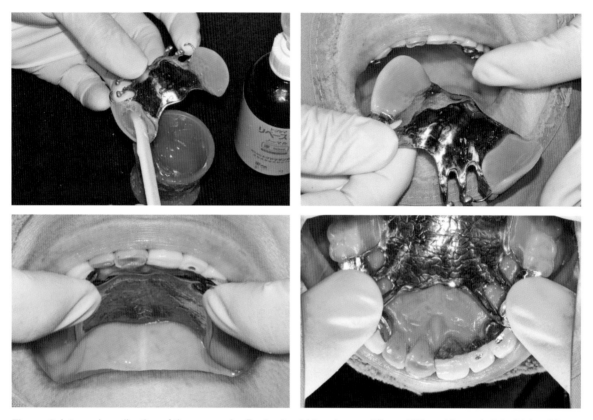

**Figure 8.** Intraoral application of the new resin. Resin should be viscous (Figure 7B) and free of air bubbles (Figure 7F).

As shown in Figure 8, the resin should not be applied if it has yet to become viscous and thick in texture. Additionally, resin should be applied slightly more than necessary, as this can help reduce the formation of air bubbles and can provide sufficient pressure as well.

**Keypoint**

Only the rests and major connectors should be pressed upon application of the reline resin. Pressure should never be put on the posterior edentulous areas. Additionally, an open-mouth technique should also be used; the patient should never bite down during the relining procedure of RPD.

An extrusion of the opposing natural teeth, as shown in Figure 9, is indicative of a denture requiring a reline. If a reline is performed properly, that is, if pressure is only applied to the appropriate pressure points, the posterior edentulous part of the metal framework will return to its original position. Then, it will once again form the desired occlusion.

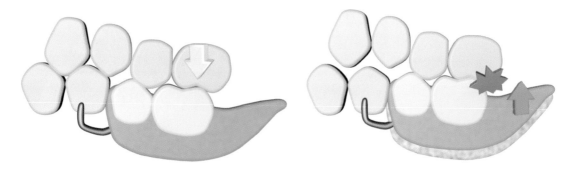

**Figure 9.** A case in which occlusal adjustments are necessary post-reline. Pressure is properly exerted only on the rests, the posterior edentulous part of the metal framework that once rotated and subsided can relocate to its original position. Then, the appropriate occlusal adjustment will be needed.

Figure 10 indicates how premature contact between the artificial and natural teeth after a reline can be adjusted. The arrows in Figure 10 show the anterior teeth disclusion due to the premature contact of

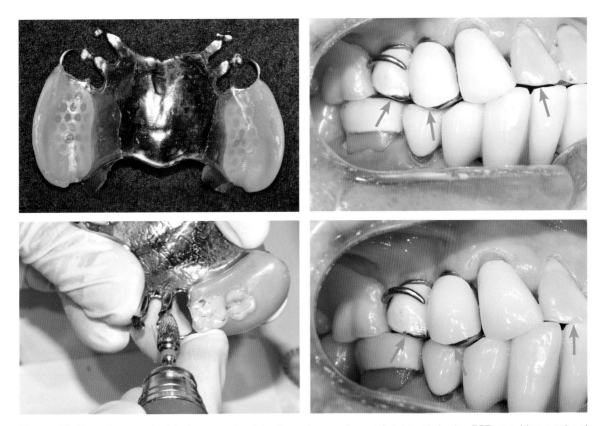

**Figure 10.** Premature contact between natural teeth and opposing artificial teeth in the RPD requiring occlusal adjustments.

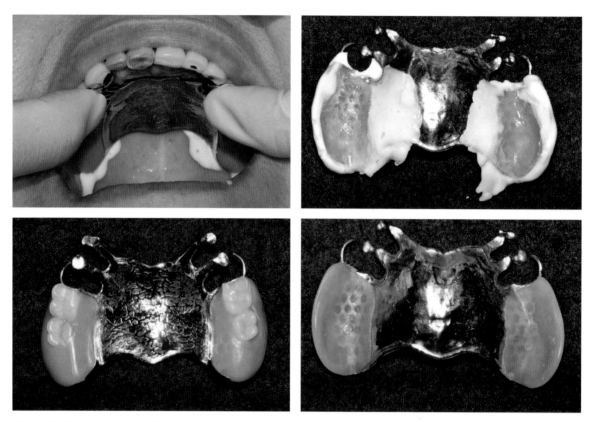

**Figure 11.** Re-examination of the denture post-reline.

the posterior artificial teeth. An immediate adjustment may be possible using a denture bur, as shown in Figure 10. However, if a great deal of adjustments must be made to the occlusion, bite registration should be taken and sent to a dental laboratory so that the appropriate changes can be made accordingly.

Regular relining is recommended because the required occlusal adjustment is often simple and the patient's adaptation to the adjusted denture is easier. In other words, periodic relining is critical for the long-term use and success of an IARPD.

The denture should be fitted to the patient to determine whether the reline was effective. With the mandible, if the rests are not lifted when the artificial teeth on the posterior edentulous area are pressed, the reline has been successfully completed. However, with the maxilla, it is difficult to determine simply based on the fit of the denture whether the reline was successful. Therefore, a fit checker or pressure indicating paste (PIP) should be used. Prior to relining, to prevent the resin from filling the tissue undercut and interrupting the path of insertion, a block-out should be performed. If occlusal adjustments are made properly as shown in Figure 10, the fit of the denture can be checked by asking the patient to bite. Figure 11 shows a well-fitted denture post-reline.

## REFERENCES

1. Da Cruz Perez LE, Machado AL, Canevarolo SV, Vergani CE, Giampaolo ET, Pavarina AC. Effect of reline material and denture base surface treatment on the impact strength of a denture base acrylic resin. Gerodontology. 2010;27:62-9.

2. Mutluay MM, Ruyter IE. Evaluation of adhesion of chairside hard relining materials to denture base polymers. J Prosthet Dent. 2005;94:445-52.

3. Takahashi JM, Machado FM, Nuñez JM, Consani RL, Mesquita MF. Relining of prosthesis with auto-polymerizing hard denture reline resins: effect of post-polymerization treatment on flexural strength. Gerodontology. 2009;26:232-6.

4. Tanoue N, Matsuda Y, Yanagida H, Matsumura H, Sawase T. Factors affecting the bond strength of denture base and reline acrylic resins to base metal materials. J Appl Oral Sci. 2013;21:320-6.

5. Tewary S, Pawashe KG. Evaluation of linear dimensional accuracy of hard chairside and laboratory heat cure reline resins at different time intervals after processing. Indian J Dent Res. 2014;25:686-91.

6. Jeong, Changmo. Atlas of Chairside Relining Technique. Shinhung International, 2001.

# The success of implant-assisted RPDs relies on establishing sufficient stability

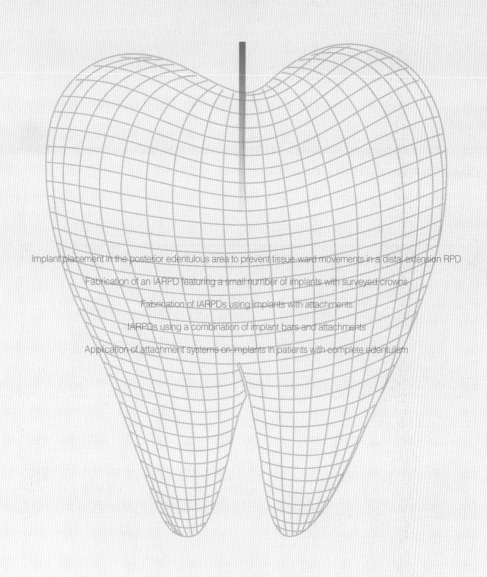

Implant placement in the posterior edentulous area to prevent tissue-ward movements in a distal extension RPD

Fabrication of an IARPD featuring a small number of implants with surveyed crowns

Fabrication of IARPDs using implants with attachments

IARPDs using a combination of implant bars and attachments

Application of attachment systems on implants in patients with complete edentulism

Chapter 4-1.

# Implant placement in the posterior edentulous area to prevent tissue-ward movements in a distal extension RPD

## Question

What are the benefits of placing implants in the posterior edentulous area in a mandibular Kennedy Class I RPD?

## Answer

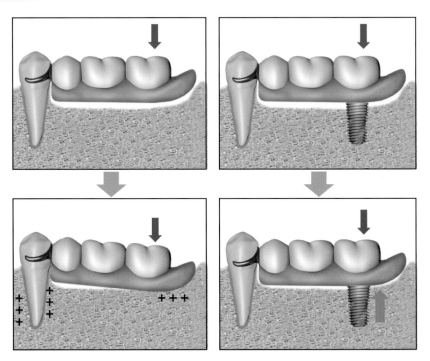

**Figure 1.** Benefits of placing implants in the posterior edentulous area of distal extension RPD. When an implant is installed in the posterior edentulous area, it can support the denture vertically, preventing the tissue-ward rotational movement of the denture.

162

Placing implants in the posterior edentulous area is what differentiates a tooth- and tissue-supported RPD (Kennedy Class I or II) from a tooth- and implant-supported RPD (Kennedy Class III). The rotation of a tooth- and tissue-supported RPD around the fulcrum line, which passes through the posterior-most abutment rests, strains the soft tissue, resulting in pain. Extreme degrees of rotational movement can also exert excessive stress on the abutment teeth. When an implant is installed in the posterior edentulous area, it can support the denture vertically, preventing the tissue-ward rotational movement of the denture base.

A survey of literature reveals that the advantages of placing implants in the posterior edentulous regions are as follows: (1) a decrease in the lateral force exerted on the residual abutment teeth (2), a decrease in the alveolar bone resorption, (3) an increase in the stability of the denture, (4) an increase in the retention when utilized with attachments and (5) an increase in the overall comfort and function. Also, some studies have reported that the combination syndrome can be prevented in patients with a maxillary complete denture and a mandibular bilateral distal extension RPD.

According to a recent systemic review by Zancope et al.(2015), most of the patients who were originally Kennedy Class I RPD wearers reported better masticatory efficiency and greater satisfaction with their Kennedy Class III RPD after installation of the implant in bilateral posterior edentulous areas. Moreover, the implant success rate was not hindered. Therefore, placing implants in bilateral distal extension cases is an effective means of limiting tissue-ward movements of the denture.

### Question

**How does placing implants in posterior edentulous areas of mandibular Kennedy Class I RPDs prevent combination syndrome in patients?**

### Answer

Combination syndrome, first identified by Ellsworth Kelly in 1972, frequently occurs in patients who wear a maxillary complete denture and a mandibular bilateral distal extension RPD. As shown in Figure 2, the distal extension RPD often loses its stability because of the resorption of the mandibular posterior alveolar ridge.

The resorption rate of the alveolar bone exponentially increases if the patient is a first-time wearer of a distal extension RPD, or if the denture is not properly relined. The resorption of the alveolar ridge can cause a tissue-ward movement of the mandibular RPD. The displacement of the maxillary and mandibular dentures results in an anteriorly positioned mandible, increased interincisal space, and extrusion of the mandibular anterior teeth. As the condition exacerbates, occlusal contact between the maxillary anterior

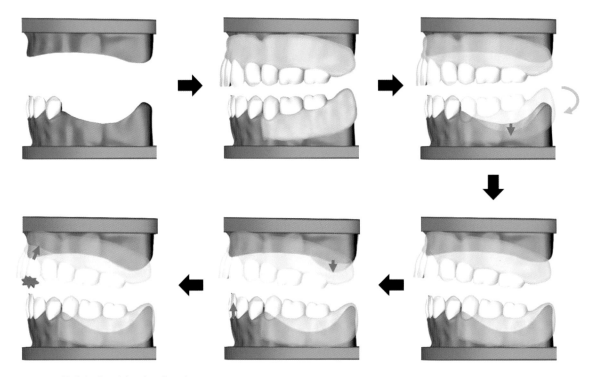

**Figure 2.** Kelly's Combination Syndrome.

artificial and mandibular natural teeth becomes excessive, and the maxillary anterior alveolar ridge gets resorbed rapidly because the remaining mandibular teeth continually thrust the maxillary denture upward. As this action continues, the maxillary denture will shift antero-superiorly, the occlusal plane will be reversed, and the vertical dimension of occlusion will be reduced. It should also be noted that the clinical signs of combination syndrome include fibrous hyperplasia with alveolar bone resorption in the anterior parts and enlargement of the tuberosity in the posterior regions of the maxilla.

Therefore, the fundamental reason of combination syndrome is alveolar bone resorption in the posterior edentulous area of the mandibular distal extension RPD. Some clinicians may recommend implant installation in the maxillary anterior region to prevent combination syndrome. However, placing implants in the mandibular posterior edentulous area, or continually relining the distal extension RPD may be more effective (Figure 3).

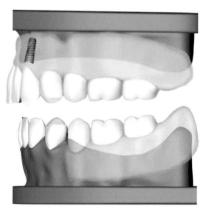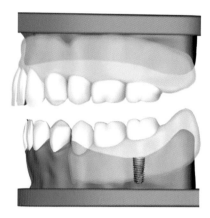

**Figure 3.** Placing implants in the mandibular posterior region is a more effective preventative measure than placing implants in the maxillary anterior region for prevention of a combination syndrome.

> **Keypoint**
>
> Implant placement in the posterior edentulous area inhibits the tissue-ward movement of a mandibular distal extension RPD and ultimately prevents combination syndrome. Nonetheless, regular relining of the RPD can also help prevent combination syndrome. Periodic maintenance of the RPD is mandatory even with implant installation since the denture can collapse posteriorly after long-term wear.

**Question**

**Which is preferable, using an attachment system or a healing abutment after implant placement in the edentulous area of a mandibular Kennedy Class I RPD?**

**Answer**

Studies have shown no significant difference between the efficacy of using healing abutments and using attachments after placing implants in the posterior edentulous areas of mandibular distal extension RPD. Therefore, the purpose of implant placement can help decide which of the two should be used. The following is a list of possible reasons for implant placement and their respective follow-up treatments.

### (1) Achieving posterior support in a distal extension RPD

A mandibular distal extension RPD base can undergo tissue-ward movement if it lacks posterior tissue support. If an implant is placed in the distal edentulous area to prevent such tissue-ward movement, healing abutments should be used for additional support. A healing abutment would come in direct contact with the denture base, allowing for potential deformations to be formed on the tooth- and implant-supported Kennedy Class III RPDs.

## (2) Enhancing retention in a distal extension RPD

If the mandibular distal extension RPD merely lacks retention, attachment systems can be applied. There are several different attachment systems available with varying degrees of rotational and vertical movements (Figure 4).

Therefore, utilizing the appropriate attachment system is important. However, most attachment systems have been produced to be used on overdentures, so they can tolerate some degree of movement, inducing less strain on the implant.

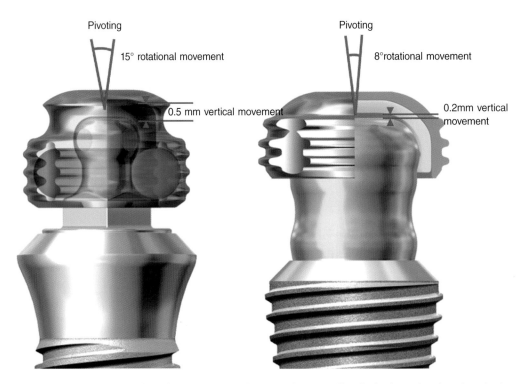

**Figure 4.** Ball-type (left) and Locator-type (right) attachments. Most attachments allow limited rotational and vertical movement. These two attachments exhibit varying ranges of movement.

This book introduces two types of attachments: ball-type and locator-type.

As shown in Figure 4, both attachment systems permit some degree of rotational and vertical movement. However, some attachments may not provide enough vertical support in the posterior edentulous area.

For example, as ball type attachments allow more vertical movement, there is a possibility of the implants securing vertical support after allowing movements for tissue support (In fact, ball attachments are not intended to provide vertical support, and they should not be used for support). The fact that attachments cannot be placed ideally according to soft tissue movement makes it challenging to predict treatment prognosis.

It is recommended that the implants be placed as close to the anterior residual teeth as possible to obtain additional retention only in the distal extension RPD. The type of attachment not only determines the level of permitted movement, but also the level of retention, stability, and support offered. Therefore, creating an IARPD that has sufficiently supportive attachments is difficult.

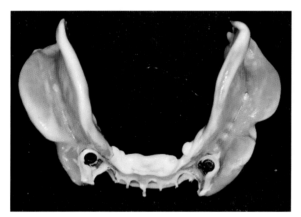 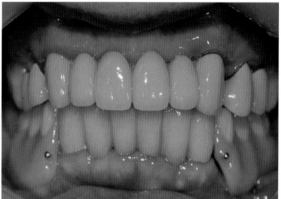

**Figure 5.** An implant placed parallel with the path of placement of the RPD will enhance the longevity of the attachment.

When an implant is placed near the anterior remaining teeth as shown in Figure 5, the implant attachment permits a slight rotational movement as detailed in Figure 4. This minimizes the rotational stress exerted on the implants as the rotational movements are made against soft tissue. Moreover, the attachment now helps with the retention of the RPD, and the use of clasps can also be omitted.

The path of insertion for the attachments should be similar to that of the RPD, which should be determined by the remaining teeth (see Chapter 2.4). If the paths of placement of the RPD and attachments are not in agreement, the RPD can crush the attachment and shorten its longevity.

## (3) Achieving posterior support and retention in a distal extension RPD

Posterior support and retention of the RPD can be established if the aforementioned considerations are put into practice.

If more than two implants are placed, their angle of insertion should be similar. Although the attachments can still be used with implants placed in different angles, having implants placed at the same angle is ideal. Studies have shown that there is a sharp decrease in the retention rate of attachments with implants placed in varying angles [Choi et al.(2017); Kim et al.(2015)]. Additionally, if both implants and attachments are placed at the same angle, not only do they last longer, but the insertion of the RPD is also easier. Admittedly, achieving ideal implant and attachment angulation is challenging, not only because there must be sufficient bone volume but also because it is a specialised skill that demands a level of mastery from the practitioner.

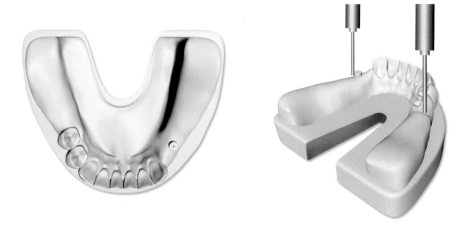

**Figure 6.** An implant placed parallel with the path of placement of the RPD will enhance the longevity of the attachment.

If at all an attachment is to be used, only those that allow very restricted vertical movement are recommended as attachments that tolerate extensive vertical movement of an IARPD. Locator attachments are preferred in that they allow for limited load relief, but magnetic attachments also seem to be an adequate choice. Healing abutments also appear to prevent tissue-ward movements of the RPD better and seem to provide greater support.

Figure 7 comprehensively encapsulates all these aspects. An RPD that relies upon implants can be considered to be similar to a traditional RPD in many respects. Overdentures retained with two implants can be categorized as implant- and tissue-supported RPDs, while overtendures retained with four implants

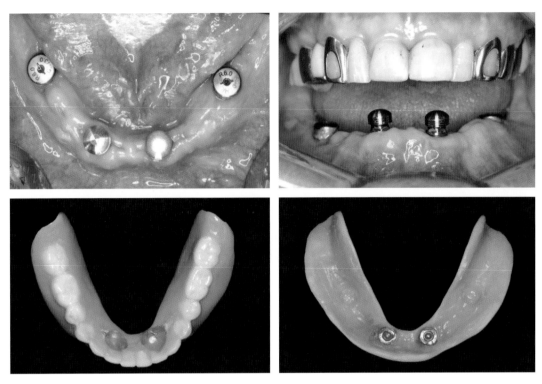

**Figure 7.** Overdenture with four implants. Only two anterior implants were given attachments, and the other two posterior implants were given healing abutments.

should be considered implant-supported RPDs if an appropriately wide aanterior-posterior spread is obtained.

Imagine a scenario in which an overdenture with four implants needs to be fabricated.

The denture would be significantly more stable if the implants have attachments as well. The implant angulation of the four implants are similar each other. This will enhance support, retention, and stability, and the denture can be categorized as an implant-supported RPD. Keep in mind that if the opposing dentition is a natural tooth, excessive occlusal force and lateral force may be transferred to the implant. However, using four attachments may be unnecessary. Disengagement of the overdenture also becomes more difficult with four locators.

Imagine, then, if only two anterior implants were given attachments, and the other two posterior implants were given healing abutments.

First, the tissue-ward movements of the denture along the fulcrum line, now formed by the mobile attachments of the two anterior implants, will be supported by the two posterior implants with healing abutments.

Second, the lateral movement of the denture can be prevented by extending the lingual flange and covering the edentulous alveolar ridge properly.

Also, the posterior implants provide support only if the lateral wall of the healing abutment is not covered by the denture base. In this way, the angle of the posterior implants becomes less important, and the implants only have to bear a vertical force. Moreover, the denture will be retained properly by the two anterior attachments.

> **Keypoint**
>
> Figure 7 indicates how posterior implants can be placed for a Kennedy Class I RPD in order to enhance posterior support. If four locators were placed here instead of two ball attachments and two healing abutments, the overdenture would be classified as a Kennedy Class III RPD, with increasing retention, support, and stability provided by the four implants.

**Question**

**Should implants be placed in the posterior area, even if this bears the greatest occlusal force? Where should implants be located in a distal extension RPD? Where should a clinician install implants?**

**Answer**

According to a clinical study conducted by Jensen et al.(2016), patient satisfaction was higher when implants were placed in the molar area than in the premolar area. Further the distance between anterior natural teeth and posterior implants, that is, the longer the edentulous region spans, the higher the risk of implant failure because the total supportive force to the implant may be increased heavily.

Besides, if the opposing dentition is a healthy natural tooth, a fixed prosthesis, or an implant fixed prosthesis, inappropriate mandibular posterior implant placement can result in an excessive occlusal force being transferred to the posterior implant and lead to implant failure.

In a retrospective study by Jensen et al.(2017), the implant success rate was 91.7%, which was higher than that seen in other studies. This may be because all other studies tested mandibular Kennedy Class I RPDs with a longer edentulous span. This study also verified the efficacy of an IARPD in mandibular Kennedy Class I cases with a high survival rate of up to 16 years and also shed light on the potential mechanical and biological side effects, and displayed better clinical results with premolar implants.

Moreover, an 8-year retrospective study conducted by Bortolini et al.(2011) concluded that nearly every patient experienced inflammation with their posterior implants. Grossmann et al.(2009) speculated that the inflammation may have resulted from the challenge of maintaining hygiene with distal implants. However, from a biomechanical perspective, the placement of the posterior implants may have brought about a transition from a Kennedy Class I RPD with several missing teeth to a Kennedy Class III IARPD with a long edentulous span. In this case, a long edentulous span will also result in a greater amount of

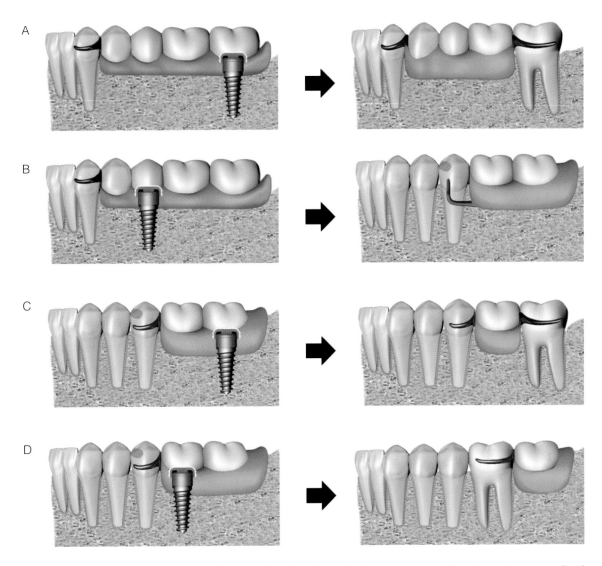

**Figure 8.** If few anterior teeth are remaining, resulting in a long edentulous span, and there is a stronger occlusal force exerted by the maxilla, then implants should be placed in the premolar area to allow for slight movements of the RPD. (A) If an implant is placed in the second molar area with a locator attachment, it acts similar to a tooth-supported RPD with surveyed crowns at the canine and second molar. (B) If the implant is placed in the second premolar area with a locator attachment, it acts similar to a tooth-tissue supported RPD with a short distal edentulous area.

stress exerted on the implants.

The experimental results obtained through Finite Element Analysis (FEA) also support this. Specifically, Cunha et al.(2008) concluded that placing implants in the premolar area is more effective than placing them in the molar area for limiting abutment displacement and stress distribution when the anterior teeth remain. In short, posteriorly placed implants can change a Kennedy Class I RPD into a tooth-implant supported Kennedy Class III RPD with a dangerously long edentulous span.

However, when implants are placed in the premolar area, the denture can be considered a Kennedy Class I RPD with a short distal extension denture base.

> **Keypoint**
>
> When the distal edentulous area is too long, due to a lack of anterior residual teeth, and the occlusal force of the opposing dentition is expected to be relatively strong, it is recommended to install the implant in the premolar area rather than in the second molar of the edentulous area, as shown in Figure 8. This will increase tissue support and prevent excessive force from being transferred to the implants. As can be seen in Figure 8, B is preferable to A, and C is preferable to D.

**Question**

**Aiming to enhance support and prevent tissue-ward movements of the RPD by using implants placed in the posterior edentulous area is reasonable in a mandibular Kennedy Class I RPD. Usually, short implants are preferred due to the lack of bone in the posterior edentulous area. This, then, raises the question of the longevity of the posterior implants, given that there may be excessive stress placed on the implants. What are the issues that must be considered?**

**Answer**

Let's review two similar clinical cases.

**Clinical case #1**(This case is from my student, and presented here with consent): Figure 9 shows a 48-year old male patient who had eight maxillary fixed implant prostheses. He wore a mandibular RPD for five years after losing all his mandibular posterior teeth, and he soon lost the rest of his mandibular anterior teeth as well.

Since he was relatively young, a fixed implant prosthesis was suggested. However, as the patient refused to receive extensive bone grafting, an IARPD was considered. The patient also wanted anterior fixed prosthesis for aesthetic reasons.

The patient was treated as shown in Figure 9, and he was satisfied with the result. Surprisingly, no side effects were seen during the 10-month follow-up.

Some questionable features can be detected from the photographs in Figure 9.

(1) A 48-year old man is expected to have strong masticatory muscles.

(2) Eight fixed implant prostheses are in the maxilla.

(3) Three implants were placed at the mandibular anterior sites, and a five-unit prosthesis was fabricated as a fixed bridge, and a surveyed bridge was used for the denture.

(4) Short implants, 6 mm in length were placed at both second molar sites, and were equipped with healing abutments.

(5) This meant that the mandibular IARPD became a Kennedy Class III RPD with a long edentulous span.

(6) For aesthetic reasons, resin clasps were fabricated on the anterior implants.

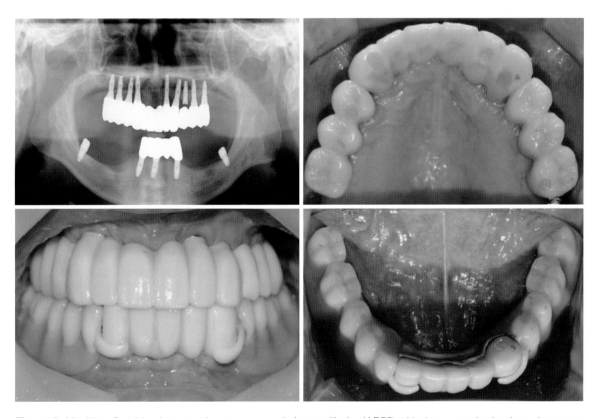

**Figure 9.** Maxillary fixed implant prostheses are used. A mandibular IARPD with three anterior implant abutments and short posterior implants with implant healing abutments is used.

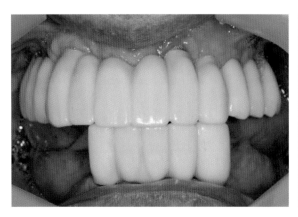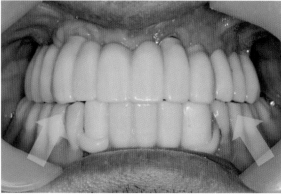

**Figure 10.** Frontal view before and after insertion of RPD. Tight contact in anterior teeth and disclusion in posterior teeth were detected.

The features listed above suggest that the treatment was mechanically unfavorable. As mentioned earlier, a Kennedy Class III RPD with a long edentulous area may put great vertical stress on the implants, predicting poor efficacy. Moreover, because the opposing dentition consisted of fixed implant prostheses, and the patient was young, the occlusal force may have been too large.

We can attribute two reasons as to why this patient did not manifest any problems. The relatively short 10-month period of time may have been a reason. Additionally, the implants may not have been as fragile as previously thought to be.

Further observation indicates that the maxillary and mandibular anterior teeth were adjusted to occlude evenly without the RPD. However, with the RPD, the posterior regions were no longer in contact.

Therefore, this patient did not have a mutually protected occlusion. A mutually protected occlusion is a natural occlusal scheme where the posterior teeth protect the anterior teeth during mastication by limiting contact between the maxillary and mandibular anterior teeth, and *vice versa*. Patients with maxillary fixed implant prostheses and a mandibular RPD with implants in the posterior edentulous area need to follow the occlusal scheme of natural dentition.

If mastication only requires the anterior teeth, even if the posterior teeth do not function properly, the patient may not experience any discomfort. However, as the posterior part of the mandibular RPD is not in contact with the opposing dentition, the long-term prognosis of this case is unpredictable and it certainly has potential problems.

**Clinical case #2:** A 68-year old female patient refused bone grafting on all ends, and only desired dental prostheses for aesthetic reasons. The treatment plan involved extraction of the upper right second molar (which had root caries) and the remaining anterior root rests in the mandible, as shown in Figure 11.

Bone grafting was necessary at the upper left lateral incisor and canine sites since the bone width was insufficient for implant placement. However, the patient refused bone grafting. An isolated abutment tooth like her upper left first premolar generally requires splinting with neighboring teeth. Therefore, a six unit bridge and maxillary RPD were planned. Four implants were placed in the mandibular anterior area instead, for aesthetic reasons. In the mandible, short implants were placed at the first molar site to

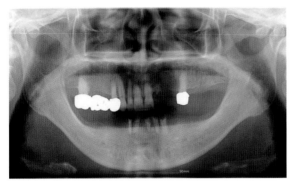 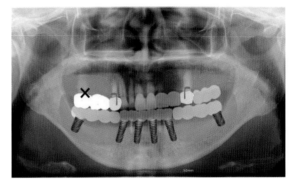

**Figure 11.** Treatment plan. In the mandible, four anterior implants and two short posterior implants would be placed. A maxillary conventional RPD would also be fabricated.

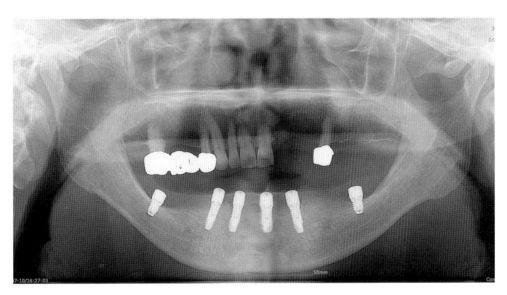

**Figure 12.** A panoramic radiograph was taken after placing six implants in the mandible. The posterior implants were installed in the molar area.

provide posterior support. Without it, the RPD would rotate about the fulcrum line and exert stress on the anterior implant-supported prostheses and edentulous areas.

Implants were placed as shown in Figure 12. Even though healing abutments, intended to provide additional support, are less sensitive to inter-implant angulation, implants should be placed as vertical to occlusal force as possible. Hirata et al.(2017) reported that implants, placed at an inclined angle to the occlusal plane, receive greater stress in proportion to the inclination of the implants.

The remaining maxillary teeth were prepared conventionally, and an impression was taken. The casts were mounted on an articulator according to the vertical dimension determined by a temporary denture as shown in Figures 13 and 14.

Customized abutments were designed and fabricated via CAD/CAM as shown in Figure 15. Figure 16 shows the setting of an abutment prosthesis. The mandibular anterior teeth were aesthetically fabricated with pink porcelain.

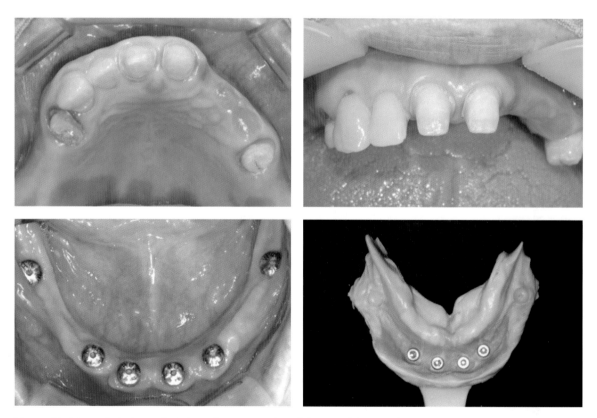

**Figure 13.** Intraoral photographs taken after preparation of the remaining maxillary teeth and implants have healed.

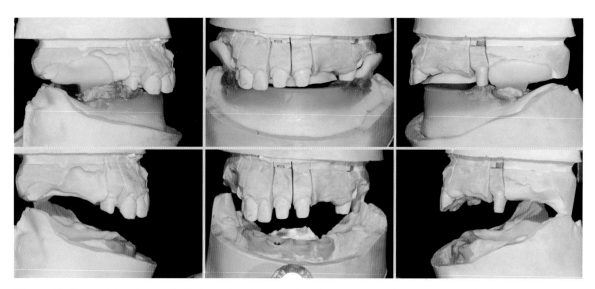

**Figure 14.** Determining the vertical dimension by mounting the temporary denture on an articulator.

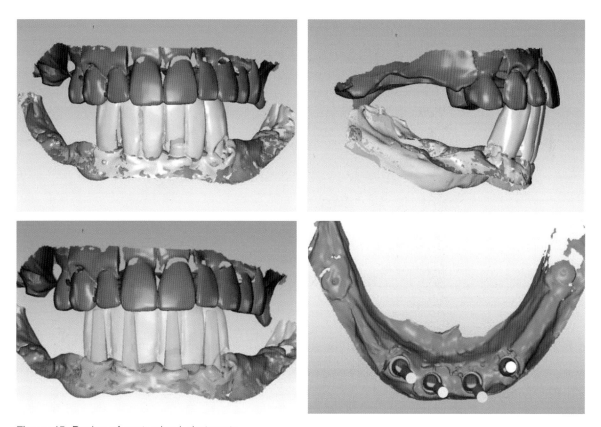

**Figure 15.** Design of customized abutments.

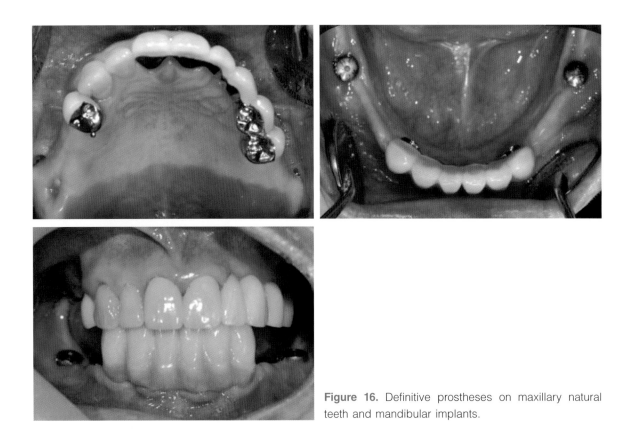

**Figure 16.** Definitive prostheses on maxillary natural teeth and mandibular implants.

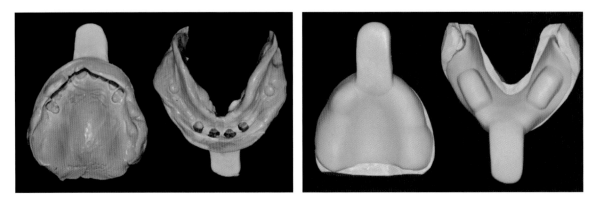

**Figure 17.** Impression for RPD taken using a customized tray.

Figure 17 shows the impression of the RPD. In the mandible, anatomical impression technique was used rather than the selective pressure impression technique because the posterior implants supported the RPD sufficiently.

Figure 18 shows the fabricated RPD. Resin clasps were added for aesthetic reasons. Resin clasps are brittle and lack elasticity, limiting their application to only RPDs that guarantee no tissue-ward movement. In this case, there was great confidence that the posterior implants would provide sufficient support and restrict

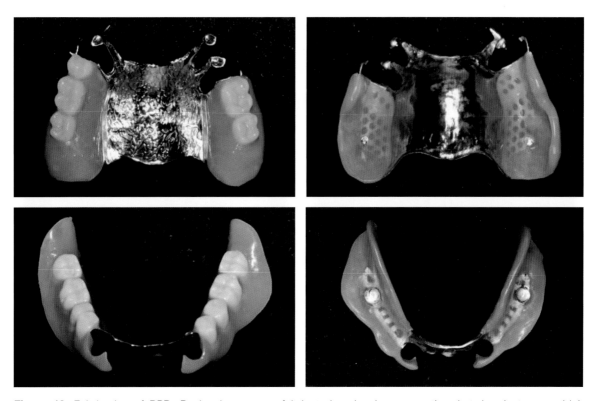

**Figure 18.** Fabrication of RPD. Resin clasps were fabricated under the assumption that the denture wouldn't rotate posteriorly toward the tissue because of sufficient implant support. Metal caps, in contact with the healing abutments, can be also considered when designing the metal framework.

rotational movement towards the tissue; therefore, the use of resin clasps was acceptable. However, when the healing abutments of the posterior implants or the tissue-side of the denture base get worn down, the denture will eventually experience tissue-ward movement. Therefore, a mandatory follow-up should be conducted every six to twelve months, and relining of the denture base or healing abutment exchange should be made when necessary. Shahmiri et al.(2017) also suggested that adding metal caps on healing abutments, created by modifying the metal framework, may reduce the chance of wear and fracture.

Figure 19 shows the application of resin clasps. If resin clasps are over-extended in the buccal region, the denture may transmit excessive stress onto the abutments or easily fracture the clasps as a result of its rotation. The resin clasps enhance retention by creating contact points between the resin and the buccal surface of abutment teeth, rather than with the undercut of the surveyed abutment teeth. Therefore, the buccal surface of the abutment teeth should also be prepared parallel to the path of insertion and removal of the RPD.

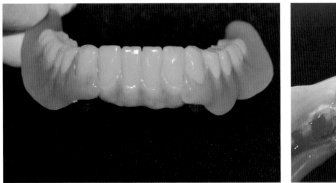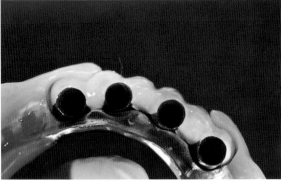

**Figure 19.** Design of resin clasps, incorporated for aesthetical reasons. Resin clasps provide retention via friction, rather than with the undercut of the surveyed abutment teeth. The clasps can be easily fractured by the excessive rotational movement of the RPD.

The RPD was delivered and adjusted to establish a tight occlusion in the posterior and a slight gap in the anterior at maximum intercuspation as shown in Figure 20. It was intended to create a mutually protected occlusion, so the anterior teeth of both arches were in contact while the posterior teeth were

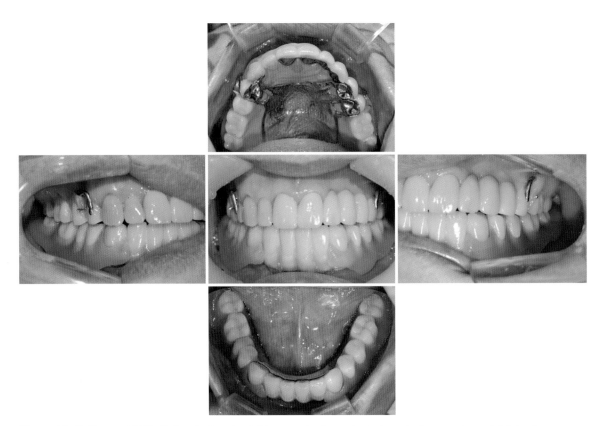

**Figure 20.** Delivery of RPD. If the denture is stable, a mutually protected occlusion can be established.

discluded during protrusive and lateral movements. Such occlusal adjustment was possible because the stability of the denture was secured by the minor connectors in contact with the abutment teeth, and also because the mandibular anterior abutment teeth with the four implants were sufficiently sturdy.

A metal cap intended to cover the top of a healing abutment can be formed by modifying the metal framework to reduce the possibility of wear and fracture. Implants can add support, but they are not designed to resist lateral forces.

As shown in Figure 21A, only the top of the healing abutment should be in contact with the metal framework or resin base; while the lateral surface of the healing abutments should be free from contact. If the healing abutment is capped completely, as shown in Figure 21B, the lateral force can be directly transferred to the implant and reduce its longevity, and this is particularly true for a short implant.

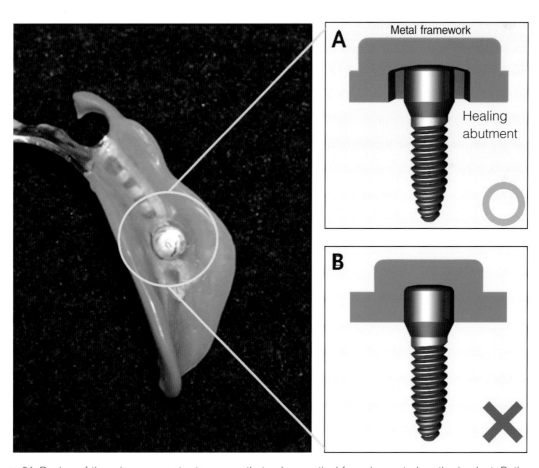

**Figure 21.** Design of the minor connector to ensure that only a vertical force is exerted on the implant. Both metal cap and metal framework placed on top of the healing abutment should transfer only vertical forces. As shown in Figure 21A, this will therefore prevent the direct loading of a lateral force.

> **Keypoint**
>
> The opposing dentition should determine how the implants are placed to provide additional posterior support. The second case required a maxillary RPD and a mandibular IARPD where implants were installed in the first molar site, which is expected to bear the greatest amount of occlusal force. In addition, the design of the metal framework was modified to minimize the lateral force exerted on the implants. A mutually protected occlusion with tight posterior contact made with maximum intercuspation was also established.

When fixed prostheses in the maxilla are significantly robust like in the first clinical case, a mandibular IARPD can be designed with posterior implants placed more anteriorly. This will allow for a slight vertical movement of the denture, and a functional impression should be taken to provide adequate tissue support.

Installing attachment systems on short implants in the mandibular posterior area is not recommended since a mandibular RPD only requires very minimal amounts of retention. Moreover, a locator attachment resists the lateral movement of implants, which may harm the implants, as shown in Figure 22. The locator attachment system is similar to a clasp on an implant abutment with a prosthesis. When it is used in the posterior edentulous area, the path of insertion and removal of the attachment and that of the RPD must be similar. Therefore, it is recommended to use healing abutments on short implants to reduce the lateral force exerted on the implants and create additional support against the vertical occlusal force. As such, it will also increase the stability and masticatory ability of the RPD.

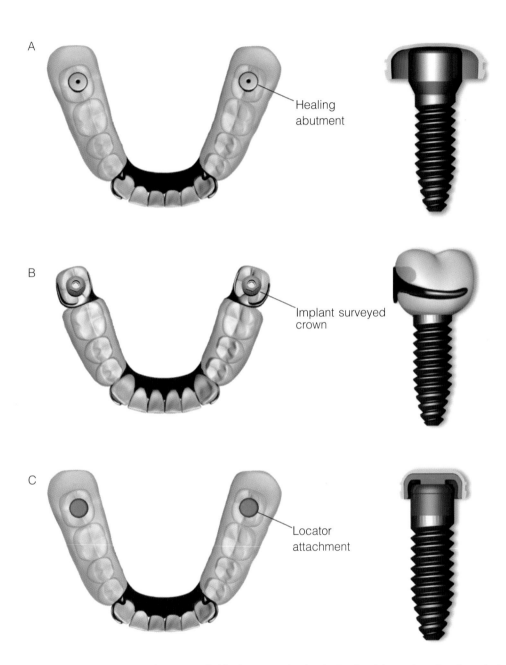

**Figure 22.** Various treatment methods are available for posterior implants. Applying only a healing abutment is recommended when a short implant is placed. Figures B and C share similar RPD structures, offering stability, support, and retention to the short implants. Compared to the prognosis of Figure A which provides only vertical support, prognoses of Figure B and C are questionable with short implants.

# REFERENCES

1.  Bortolini S, Natali A, Franchi M, Coggiola A, Consolo U. Implant-retained removable partial dentures: an 8-year retrospective study. J Prosthodont. 2011;20:168.172.

2.  Choi JW, Bae JH, Jeong CM, Huh JB. Retention and wear behaviors of two implant overdenture stud-type attachments at different implant angulations. J Prosthet Dent. 201;117:628-635.

3.  Cunha LD, Pellizzer EP, Verri FR, Pereira JA. Evaluation of the influence of location of osseointegrated implants associated with mandibular removable partial dentures. Implant Dent. 2008;17:278-87.

4.  Derks J, Schaller D, Hakansson J, Wennstrom JL, Tomasi C, Berglundh T. Effectiveness of implant therapy analyzed in a Swedish population: prevalence of peri-implantitis. J Dent Res. 2016;95:43-49.

5.  Grossmann Y, Nissan J, Levin L. Clinical effectiveness of implant-supported removable partial dentures: a review of the literature and retrospective case evaluation. J Oral Maxillofac Surg 2009;67:1941-1946.

6.  Hirata K, Takahashi T, Tomita A, Gonda T, Maeda Y. Influence of Abutment Angle on Implant Strain When Supporting a Distal Extension Removable Partial Dental Prosthesis: An in Vitro Study. Int J Prosthodont. 2017;30:51-53.

7.  Jacob RF, King GE. Partial Denture Framework Design for Bone-Grafted Mandibles Restored with Osseointegrated Implants. Journal of Prosthodontics. 1995;4:6-10.

8.  Jensen C, Meijer HJA, Raghoebar GM, Kerdijk W, Cune MS. Implant-supported removable partial dentures in the mandible: A 3-16-year retrospective study. J Prosthodont Res. 2017;61:98-105.

9.  Jensen C, Raghoebar GM, Kerdijk W, Meijer HJ, Cune MS. Implant-supported mandibular removable partial dentures; patient-based outcome measures in relation to implant position. Journal of Dentistry. 2016;25:92-98.

10. Kelly E. Changes caused by a mandibular removable partial denture opposing a maxillary complete denture. The Journal of Prosthetic Dentistry. 1972;27:140-150.

11. Keltjens HM, Kayser AF, Hertel R, Battistuzzi PG. Distal extension removable partial dentures supported by implants and residual teeth: considerations and case reports. International Journal of Oral & Maxillofacial Implants. 1993;8:208-213.

12. Kim SM, Choi JW, Jeon YC, Jeong CM, Yun MJ, Lee SH, Huh JB. Comparison of changes in retentive force of three stud attachments for implant overdentures. J Adv Prosthodont. 2015;7:303-311.

13. Mijiritsky E, Lorean A, Mazor Z, Levin L. Implant tooth supported removable partial denture with at least 15-year longterm follow-up. Clin Implant Dent Relat Res. 2015;17:917-922.

14. Mitrani R, Brudvik JS, Phillips KM. Posterior implants for distal extension removable prostheses: a retrospective study. International Journal of Periodontics & Restorative Dentistry. 2003;23:353-359.

15. Pellizzer EP, Verri FR, Falcon-Antenucci RM, Goiato MC, Gennari Filho H. Evaluation of different retention systems on a distal extension removable partial denture associated with an osseointegrated implant. J Craniofac Surg.

2010;21:727-34.

16. Saunders TR. The maxillary complete denture opposing the mandibular bilateral distal-extension partial denture: treatment considerations. The Journal of Prosthetic Dentistry. 1979;41:124-128.

17. Shahmiri R, Das R. Finite element analysis of implant-assisted removable partial dentures: Framework design considerations. J Prosthet Dent. 2017;118:177-186.

18. Wismeijer D, Tawse-Smith A, Payne AG. Multicentre prospective evaluation of implant-assisted mandibular bilateral distal extension removable partial dentures: patient satisfaction. Clin Oral Implants Res. 2013;24:20-27.

19. Zancope K, Abrao GM, Karam FK, Neves FD. Placement of a distal implant to convert a mandibular removable Kennedy Class I to an implant-supported partial removable Class III dental prosthesis: A systematic review. J Prosthet Dent. 2015;113:528-33.

Chapter 4-2.

# Fabrication of an IARPD featuring a small number of implants with surveyed crowns

This chapter discusses a clinical situation where implants with surveyed crowns directly provide the RPD with additional retention, stability, and support. Admittedly, this type of treatment still requires more research to prove its efficacy. However, it is still believed to be a viable option. Transitioning from a tooth-tissue supported Kennedy Class I or II RPD to a Kennedy Class III RPD can simplify treatment as well as increase patient satisfaction, but the long-term prognosis remains disputable. Examining the strength of the occlusal force is necessary; the opposing dentition and bone volume at the desired implant placement site can help predict the amount of force to be exerted upon the implant.

### Question

**What needs to be taken into consideration before fabricating an IARPD?**

### Answer

Listed below are a variety of scenarios and the appropriate factors to be considered for each scenario.

### 1. Cases that do not require the correction of the occlusal plane

Patients with inadequate occlusal planes, such as those with an eruption of residual teeth, are not suitable for an IARPD that uses implant surveyed crowns as abutments. Specifically, patients with the combination syndrome, which results in the extrusion of residual teeth or large alveolar bone resorption of the opposite jaw, require a correction of the occlusal plane and the use of other attachment systems rather than surveyed crowns.

In the following case, the fabrication of the maxillary and mandibular IARPD without having to correct the occlusal plane was possible because neither an extrusion of the right upper residual teeth nor severe mandibular bone resorption was observed (Figures 1-6).

In this case, the IARPDs were fabricated without having to correct the occlusal plane because the residual abutments did not experience excessive lateral force during eccentric movement and showed no significant resorption of the mandibular bone. However, if the occlusal plane was inadequate, or the extruded tooth interfered with lateral movement, the harmful lateral force could be transferred directly to the implant with surveyed crowns. The existing occlusal plane should be examined carefully to create a proper, balanced occlusion.

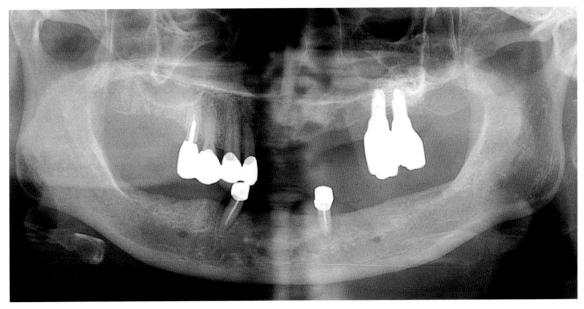

**Figure 1.** Panoramic radiograph. In the left upper molar area, two implant surveyed crowns that form a proper occlusal plane with the right residual teeth are shown. The lower residual teeth were to be extracted due to severe mobility.

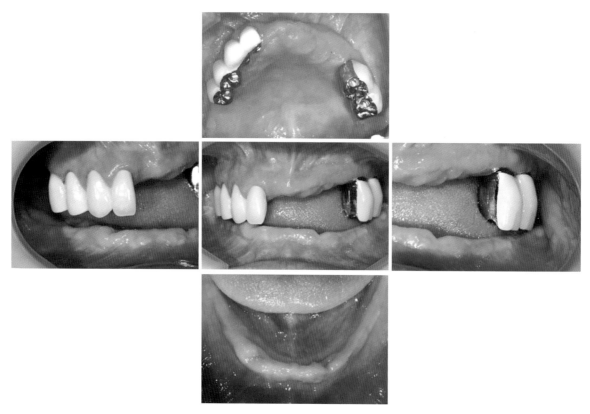

**Figure 2.** After extraction of lower residual teeth. The maxillary abutments showed no extrusion or imbalance, and the mandibular alveolar ridge showed no severe vertical bone resorption. Therefore, the existing occlusal plane was to be left untouched, and both upper and lower IARPDs were to be fabricated.

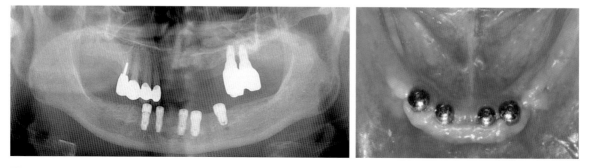

**Figure 3.** Post-implant placement in the mandible. The implant installed at the left first premolar area failed.

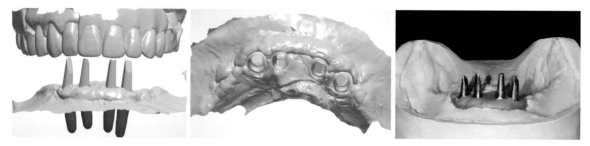

**Figure 4.** Fabrication of customized abutments.

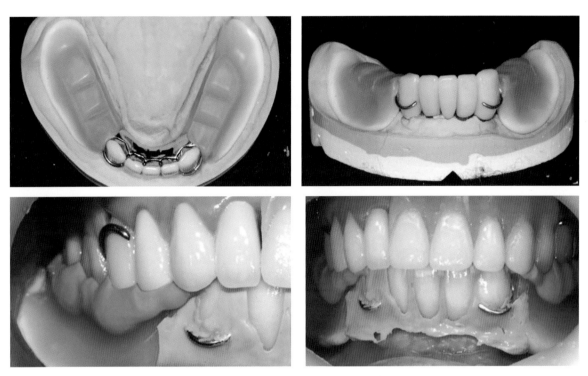

**Figure 5.** Bite registration with a stable occlusal rim.

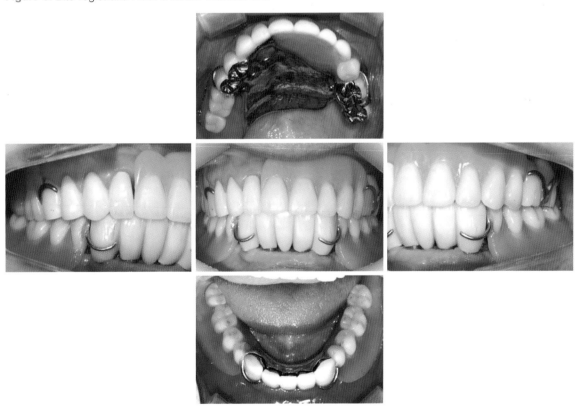

**Figure 6.** Delivery of the maxillary and mandibular IARPD's: A maxillary IARPD with implant surveyed crowns at the left first and second molar sites and a mandibular IARPD with a five-unit implant surveyed crown bridge in the anterior were fabricated.

## 2. Cases with improper restorable space for the installation of an implant surveyed crown

Implants with surveyed crowns require at least 4 mm of restorable space. Otherwise, it is difficult to fabricate the prosthesis itself. In cases where the restorable space is too large, however, a treatment with implant surveyed crowns is inappropriate.

There are three reasons for this:

First, attachments reduce the lateral force on the implant by lowering the point of action of the

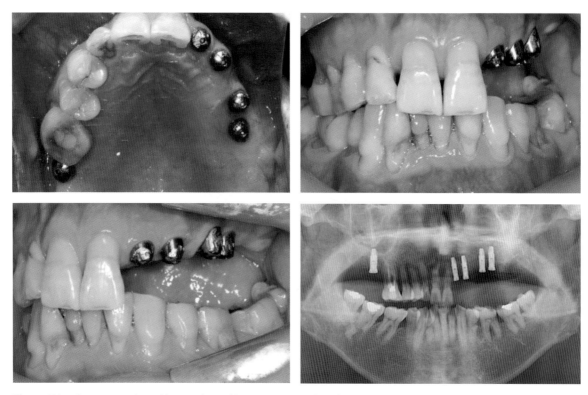

**Figure 7.** Implants were placed in a patient with severe resorption of maxillary alveolar bone without full consideration of the final prostheses. Implant insertion path is tilted labially, and a significant amount of vertical restorable space is shown.

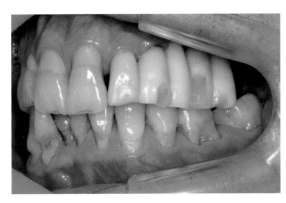
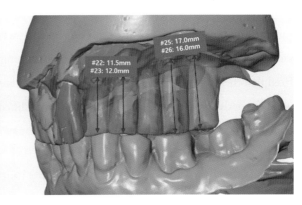

**Figure 8.** Assessment of fixed implant prostheses by temporary prostheses. The long crown length creates aesthetic and maintenance concerns.

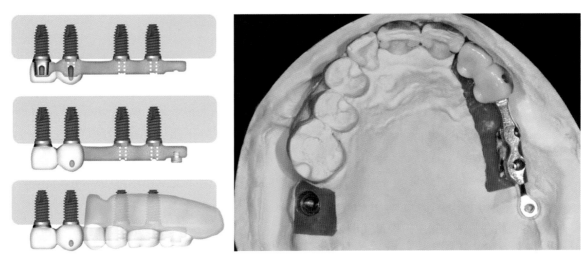

**Figure 9.** Combined treatment of implant surveyed crowns and bar attachments with locator attachments.

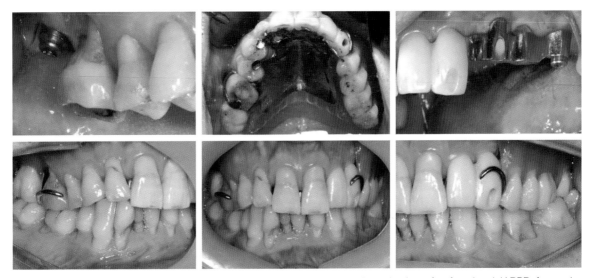

**Figure 10.** Recovery of anterior teeth to solve aesthetic problems and production of a functional IARPD for easier maintenance. Since the residual natural teeth have periodontitis resulting in slight mobility, support was increased with a full palatal coverage major connector, and this made it easier to repair in the later extraction of some residual teeth.

191

force. Second, the height of implant surveyed crown may be too tall and result in aesthetic concerns, whereas attachments are aesthetically more gratifying. Third, bar attachments require more space than fixed prostheses. Therefore, if the restorable space is large, a robust implant bar attachment should be used with the IARPD. Figures 7 to 10 show the modified methods to treat cases of severe bone resorption and the combined application of surveyed prostheses and bar attachments.

### 3. Cases in which implants can be installed at ideal sites for a stable IARPD

To ensure the stability of an IARPD, the placement of the implant should be determined after carefully considering the location of the fulcrum line and the mobility of the denture. In addition, the condition of the alveolar bone should also be taken into consideration.

### 4. Cases in which the position of the artificial teeth and those of the implants are buccolingually in concordance.

When an implant surveyed crown is used as an abutment, the position of the prosthesis depends on the implantation site. On the other hand, the arrangement of the artificial teeth in the IARPD is determined by the remaining natural teeth, the positioning of the opposing dentition, as well as the aesthetic concerns regarding the anterior teeth. In other words, the RPD design should ensure that the implant surveyed crowns and the artificial teeth create the desired occlusion.

Let us consider a scenario where an implant is located more lingually than the artificial tooth by a

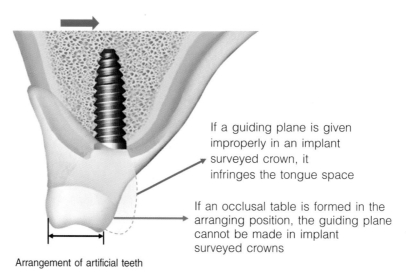

If a guiding plane is given improperly in an implant surveyed crown, it infringes the tongue space

If an occlusal table is formed in the arranging position, the guiding plane cannot be made in implant surveyed crowns

Arrangement of artificial teeth

**Figure 11.** The errors due to the difference between arrangement of artificial teeth and inserted implant position. It is preferable to use attachments instead of surveyed crown in this case.

few millimeters. If the occlusal surface of the implant surveyed crown is aligned only with the artificial tooth, the oblique lingual guiding plane will cause a large lateral force to be exerted on the implant during occlusion (Figure 11). The guiding plane should align with the path of insertion. Therefore, if the aforementioned conditions cannot be obtained, it is preferable to use attachments instead, since attachments cannot be affected by the artificial tooth arrangement and buccolingual positioning of the implants in an IARPD.

### 5. Cases in which the angle of the implant and the path of insertion of the IARPD are not parallel.

When using attachments, including the locator attachment system, it is necessary to match the path of insertion of the IARPD with the angle of the implant installation as much as possible. If they are not parallel, the female part of the locator quickly gets worn down, leading to reduced retention (Figure 12). If the angle of insertion of the implants exceeds the permitted angular range of an attachment, it cannot be applied.

However, implant surveyed crowns can be used in place of attachments, by altering their shapes, even if the angle is significantly misaligned with the residual natural teeth.

One of the great benefits of using implant surveyed crowns as RPD abutments is that they can be used as long as the guiding plane is prepared appropriately according to the path of insertion of the IARPD.

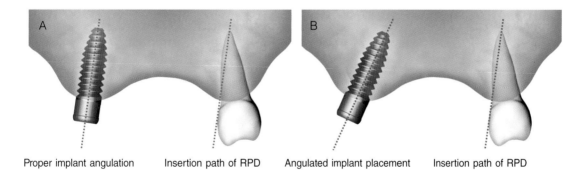

Proper implant angulation    Insertion path of RPD          Angulated implant placement    Insertion path of RPD

**Figure 12.** When using an attachment system, the path of insertion of the RPD and the angle of implantation must be parallel, as shown in A. Therefore, if the angular difference is large as in B, attachment systems can not be used.

### 6. Cases in which the use of clasps is acceptable

Treatment using implant surveyed crowns as abutments bring about aesthetic concerns because of the clasps that need to be added. If patients refuse to have clasps, then attachments should be used instead of implant surveyed crowns because the former yields higher patient satisfaction in terms of aesthetics.

**What is the difference between an implant-retained RPD and an implant-assisted RPD?**

Several studies, including those by Yeung et al.(2014), Shahmiri et al.(2014), Gharehchani et al.(2013), and Wismeijer et al.(2013), have reported the differences between implant-retained RPDs and implant-assisted RPDs (IARPD). Implant-assisted RPDs are dentures that have additional stability, retention, and vertical support provided by the installed implants. Unfortunately, however, research has shown that the lateral forces acting directly on the implants of these IARPDs could result in potential problems.

The distinction between implant-retained RPDs and implant-assisted RPDs, typically determined by the placement site of the implant and type of attachment used, sometimes becomes unclear, as shown in Figure 13. Therefore, the identity of an RPD can also be determined with a comprehensive understanding of its design as well as of the characteristics of the chosen attachment systems. Visualizing the movement of the RPD and predicting the different forces acting upon the abutment teeth and implants may also help in categorization.

Let us consider two different treatment plans: one with a locator attachment system that allows little vertical and horizontal movements, and the other with a ball attachment system that permits gross movements (Locator is a brand name but used here for convenience). Figure 13A, displays a tissue-supported Kennedy Class I RPD fitted for a patient with six anterior remaining teeth and implants and locator attachments placed at the bilateral premolar sites. The locator attachments allow for a certain range of rotational movement, including the tissue-ward movement by the posterior part of the RPD. For example, 1 mm of subsidence in the molar area results in less down ward displacement in the first premolar area. In addition, as the locators can tolerate slight rotational movement, the implants placed on the premolar site also allow a certain level of denture movement, and thus the lateral force transferred to the implants will be less.

If implants are placed in the posterior edentulous area, the force will be transferred to the attachments rather than to the soft tissue, as shown in Figure 13B. This type of denture can be classified as a Kennedy Class III RPD. Specifically, when a locator type is used, stability can be achieved through tight coupling between the female part and the lateral wall of the male part of the attachment. This provides retenion, posterior support, and stability, but may also exert a significant amount of external force on the implant itself.

Figure 13C describes a ball attachment system with a full range of movement, both vertically and horizontally. In this case, when the edentulous part of the RPD is pressed, the entire vertical load will be transferred to the soft tissue since the attachment does not provide any vertical support. In addition, a structure that permits horizontal movement cannot ensure stability. It only enhances the retention of

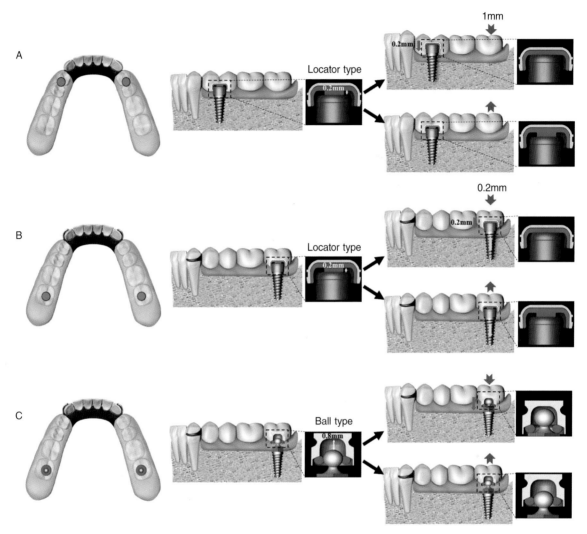

**Figure 13.** Categorizing various RPDs: implant-retained RPD and implant-assisted RPD combined with implant attachments. (A) Implants and Locators placed at the bilateral premolar sites, (B) Implants and Locators placed at the bilateral second molar sites, (C) Implants and ball attachments placed at the bilateral second molar sites. Locator attachment system offers vertical support and allows for slight vertical movements of by the RPD base. In contast, the ball attachment system doesn't provide much vertical support. Both attachments allow denture movement.

the denture, and thus this type can be classified as an implant-retained RPD. It is important, then, to take functional impressions and add stress breaker type direct retainers (like wrought wire clasps) onto the canines.

---

**Keypoint**

The difference between an implant retained RPD and an implant-assisted RPD relies not on the location of implant, but rather on the type of attachment system.

---

## Question

**What are the advantages and disadvantages of an implant-assisted RPD? What should be considered?**

## Answer

Mijiritsky (2007) reported better masticatory efficiency and patient satisfaction with an implant-assisted RPD, in which implants were used as abutments to provide retention, support, and stability. Other studies also revealed additional potential benefits, including tooth protection, decreased residual bone resorption, and increased cost reduction.

Eom et al.(2017) performed a 3-dimensional finite element analysis (FEA) on a unilaterally designed tooth- supported RPD and an implant- supported RPD in 2016. The study revealed that a substantial amount of stress was exerted on the implants. The study emphasized the importance of choosing the appropriate number and positioning of implants when designing the RPD. Numerous implants, splinted prostheses, and maximum coverage of the posterior edentulous area in the distal extension RPD can help prevent prosthesis fractures, peri-implant bone resorption, and implant failure. The study also concluded that fabricating a Kennedy class I or II implant tissue-supported RPD with anteriorly positioned implants may be preferable to an IARPD in which stress is offloaded onto the implants directly.

A Kennedy class I RPD with only six anterior remaining teeth requires a different treatment than that of an RPD of a patient with anterior and premolar teeth. A long edentulous span in a Kennedy Class III RPD transfers forces onto the canine and implant surveyed crown in the molar area. A treatment plan should be developed based on the opposing dentition and natural teeth abutments.

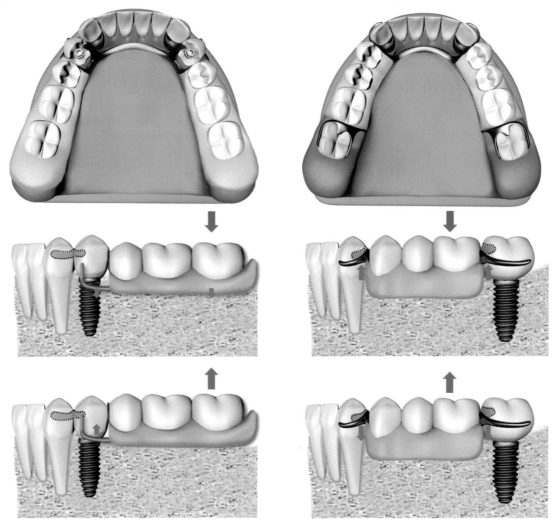

**Figure 14.** Application of an implant- surveyed crown on a Kennedy class I RPD. With six anterior teeth remaining, determining the location of the implant installation is particularly important; if they are placed on the premolar area, the denture will be classified as a Kennedy class I RPD, and if the implants are placed in the molar area, the denture will be classified as a Kennedy class III RPD.

**Question**

**In patients who only have anterior teeth remaining, where should the implants with surveyed crowns be placed?**

**Answer**

The clinical case below will be used as an example to illustrate what factors should be taken into

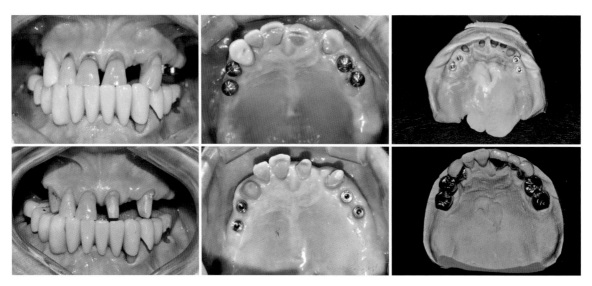

**Figure 15.** A 73-year old female with great mobility in the anterior teeth of the maxilla resulting from long-term masticatory activity with the remaining teeth.

consideration when determining the placement of implants.

The following case details a 73-year old female patient, who is on medication for diabetes and hypertension. As shown in Figure 15, the upper left lateral incisor was missing, and the remaining teeth presented slight mobility.

First, the mandibular opposing dentition, composed of fixed prostheses on natural teeth abutments, was evaluated. The patient expressed no discomfort, so she did not want retreatment. Second, it was evident that nearly half of the alveolar bone around the remaining anterior teeth of the maxilla was resorbed. Although the anterior teeth showed slight mobility as a result of mastication, extraction did not seem necessary. It was clear that the issue with mobility in the anterior teeth would be resolved once posterior support was secured.

The patient agreed to receive two implants on each side and was told that fixed prostheses would be possible with implant placement in the premolar and molar areas. However, her preexisting health conditions prevented her from getting a bone graft. Therefore, the two implants were installed in the premolar area without bone grafting. Then, the right canine along with the left incisor and left canine were restored with a 3-unit bridge to function as RPD abutments and cingulum rests were created for both canines.

The RPD was fabricated with implant surveyed crowns as shown in Figures 16 and 17. The mesial rests were designed on the implant surveyed crowns, and the wrought-wire clasps were designed to allow for a

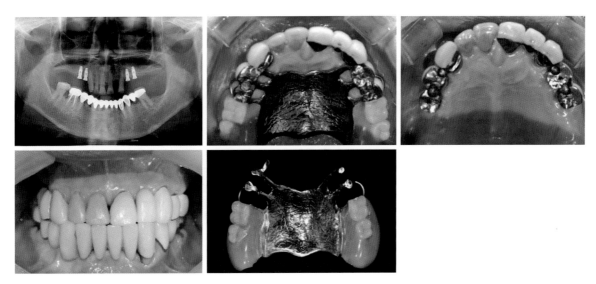

**Figure 16.** Fabrication of an RPD using two fixed implant prostheses as abutments on the premolar sites on each side.

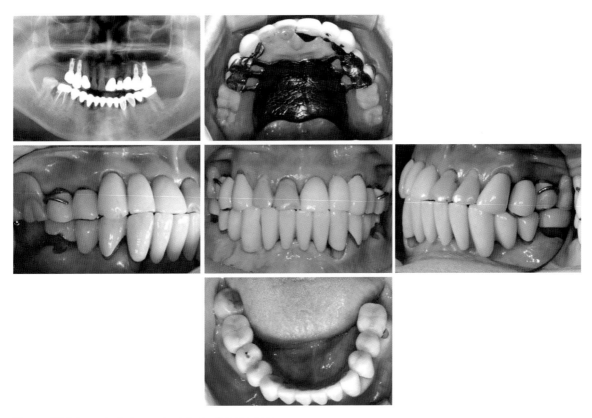

**Figure 17.** Intraoral photographs taken after 5 years.

limited degree of tissue-ward movement during mastication in the posterior area. The artificial teeth were made to have close contact, while the anterior teeth were made to have light contact (a sheet of shim stock could be slipped through the contact point). Also, canine guidance was successfully established. Every six months, the occlusion and fit of the RPD were checked. Relining of the denture base was performed twice within the past five years.

The patient reported no discomfort at the 5-year follow-up. The alveolar bone level in the anterior teeth was stable, and the anterior teeth showed no mobility. The condition of the implants was stable as well.

### Keypoint

Fixed implant prostheses might have resulted in greater patient satisfaction. However, additional bone grafting would have been necessary, and alveolar bone resorption would have increased the crown length, leading to difficulty in oral hygiene maintenance and poor prognosis of the implants. In the maxilla, at least two implants should be splinted at a minimum, and the patient should be instructed to wear the RPD at all times, except when sleeping. A common misconception is that distal extension RPD would create patient discomfort because a greater force would be transferred to the RPD and supporting tissue. However, the application of wrought-wire clasps and mesial rests would contribute to the reduction of stress on implants by tolerating the functional movement of the RPD during mastication.

### Question

**When is it most beneficial to use implant surveyed crowns as RPD abutments if two implants are to be placed in the maxilla?**

### Answer

Even with just two implants, the RPD can still be successful if there is sufficient unilateral edentulous space.

A 72-year old female patient with severe vertical bone resorption in the maxillary right quadrant came in wearing an RPD.

As shown in Figure 18, the lower right third molar with first degree mobility was used as an abutment tooth for a mandibular Kennedy Class II RPD. In the maxilla, most of the teeth in the left quadrant remained in acceptable condition.

In this case, placing the implants in the upper right first and second molar areas could create a tooth-

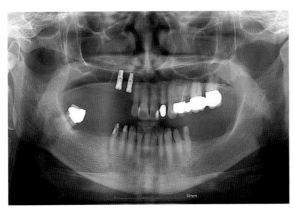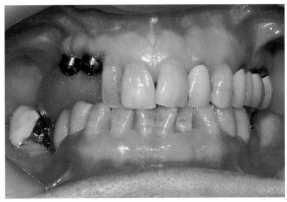

**Figure 18.** A case showing implants being placed at the canine and premolar sites, with the posterior teeth remaining intact unilaterally.

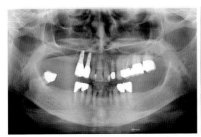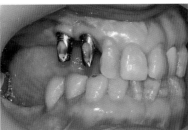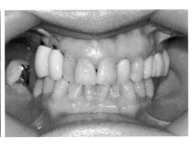

**Figure 19.** Delivery of implant surveyed crowns for the maxillary right canine and first premolar.

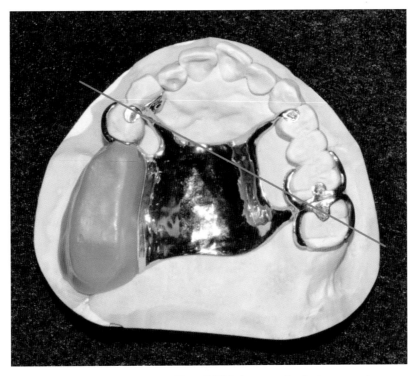

**Figure 20.** Design of a Kennedy Class II RPD that uses implant surveyed crowns on the upper right canine and first premolar.

supported RPD, but the lingual rest could not be formed due to linguoversion of the upper right lateral incisor. What is more, even if the lingual rest could be fabricated appropriately, the denture would have a long edentulous span and fail to evenly distribute forces, resulting in a large amount of stress concentrated on the lateral incisor or posterior implants. Therefore, implants were installed at the right canine and first premolar area to be restored with surveyed crowns.

In order to avoid bone grafting, the implants were intentionally placed in the maxillary right canine and first premolar area where the alveolar bone was sufficient.

When the alveolar bone shows severe vertical resorption, the margin of the porcelain crown need not be subgingival. If the gingiva around the tooth is not exposed while speaking or smiling, an intentional supragingival margin can be created instead, which will also help the patient to maintain hygiene. The preparation of a proper undercut and precise mesial rest on the upper right first premolar is important. Besides, the positioning of the minor connectors and the guiding plane should exactly match with the RPD's path of insertion. A well-prepared abutment crown offers enhanced retention and a refined path of insertion, reducing the chances of repetitive disengagement of the cement-retained implant bridge restoration. An excessive undercut or a poorly prepared path of insertion may result in an extremely tight fit.

The upper right first premolar implant formed the fulcrum line with the upper left second molar, allowing for the necessary rotational movement of the RPD, and the upper left first premolar was not equipped with a clasp to reduce the stress caused by such rotational movements. Also, a rest was created for the upper left first premolar to act as an indirect retainer for the RPD. This is meant to evenly distribute vertical support and will contribute to the retention of the clasp from the posterior-most abutment teeth. As splinted healthy posterior teeth can provide sufficient stability to the RPD, the embrasure clasp was designed to fit into the maxillary left posterior teeth. The goal was to minimize the movement of the RPD so that less stress would be exerted on the implant abutment.

A stable RPD was fabricated using two implant-surveyed crowns, as shown in Figure 21. During maximum intercuspation, the artificial teeth were occluded in tight contact as a number of natural teeth and implants were eligible for the natural occlusal scheme. If the posterior part of the RPD does not offer sufficient support, the patient may masticate with the right mandibular abutment teeth and maxillary implant surveyed crowns, putting great strain on the implant abutments. Therefore, the choice of an occlusal scheme requires attention.

The lower right third molar presented horizontal mobility, but it was thought to provide sufficient support. Therefore, a rest was designed without a clasp in the RPD. A Kennedy Class I RPD was designed

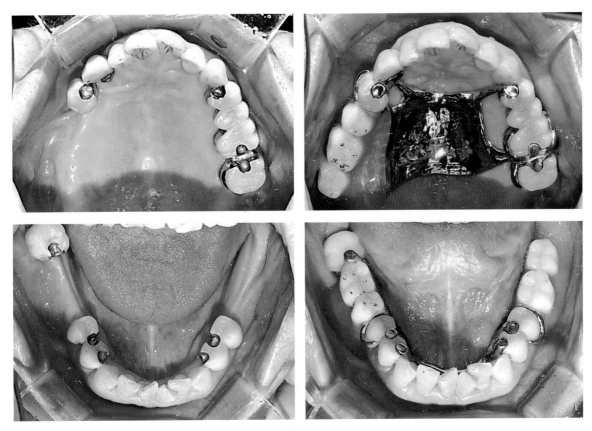

**Figure 21.** Delivery of the maxillary and mandibular RPD

so that the mandibular RPD could be altered in case the lower-right third molar was to be extracted (see Chapter 3.2).

**Question**

**Can two implants be placed in the maxillary posterior area? What patient-related factors must be considered?**

**Answer**

A clinician must consider the following:

(1) Would the RPD become a tooth-supported RPD with a long edentulous span, if the two implants were to be installed in the maxillary posterior area?

(2) Can rest seats be created and supported by the remaining anterior teeth?

(3) What is the condition of the opposing dentition? Will the long edentulous span exert excessive

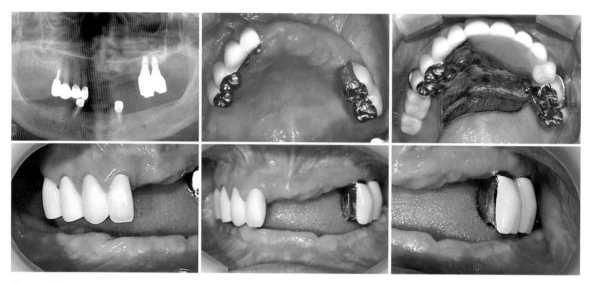

**Figure 22.** A clinical case in which the RPD was fabricated using two implant surveyed crowns in the posterior area of the maxilla.

stress on the abutment teeth?

(4) If implants with elongated crowns were to be used in patients with severe vertical bone resorption in the posterior regions, how will that affect maintenance of hygiene?

Let us consider the following clinical case (Figure 22).

A 72-year old female patient received two implants in the left maxillary area and a new RPD was fabricated. After the treatment, she felt comfortable with the new maxillary RPD.

The remaining teeth existed only on one side of the arch, but the implants placed on the other edentulous side enhanced the support and stability of the RPD. However, the RPD had a significantly long edentulous span that could have transferred excessive force onto the abutment teeth and implants, which were bearing the entire support of the denture. However, because the patient's opposing dentition was in a edentulous state, the masticatory force of the mandibular denture did not seem to cause any serious problems. As previously mentioned, the location of the implant installation depends on the condition of the opposing dentition and the span of the edentulous area. The challenge presented by this case was the aggravating condition of the mandible. Placing the implant in the left maxillary posterior region enhanced the masticatory force transferred to the posterior area. Therefore, periodic relining and proper occlusal adjustments are necessary to prevent the rotational movements of the RPD and to protect the abutments. Also, the patient may now be vulnerable to developing peri-implantitis. The patient exhibited vertical bone resorption, therefore the crown prostheses were elongated. Maintenance of hygiene is difficult and food may get stuck near the cervical region of the prostheses.

Placing the implants in the canine and premolar could have made hygiene maintenance easier on the patient, and periodic relining could have created a more balanced tooth (implant) and tissue-supported RPD.

**If the patient presents severe bone resorption in the posterior region of the mandible, where should the implants be installed?**

The treatment plans for the mandible and maxilla are quite similar. However, when the anterior teeth in the mandible remain and the alveolar bone is still in a moderate condition, a mandibular RPD may be fabricated using only one implant surveyed crown, unlike in a maxillary RPD, where two implants must be placed next to each other and splinted together.

The following clinical cases illustrate this point.

**Case #1:** A 63-year old female patient experienced constant pain in the left mandibular posterior edentulous area ever since she had started wearing her mandibular RPD. She wanted to get it replaced, adding implants with fixed prostheses. An extensive bone graft was necessary due to severe bone resorption. Therefore, two implants were to be placed at the lower-left first and second premolar site without a bone graft, as the patient had a complete denture for the maxilla. If the patient had sufficient bone levels for the placement of short implants, they would have been placed in the posterior-most area, connected to healing abutments for support. However, this was not the case for this patient.

The symmetry between the left and right sides can be achieved by placing implants at the lower-left first and second premolar sites as shown in Figure 23. The implant placement can also offer natural teeth and implant-surveyed crowns additional support by adding a mesial rest, an indirect retainer, and a clasp that would allow for some tissue-ward movement in the posterior edentulous area. The posterior edentulous area would also enhance support, so a stable RPD was predicted.

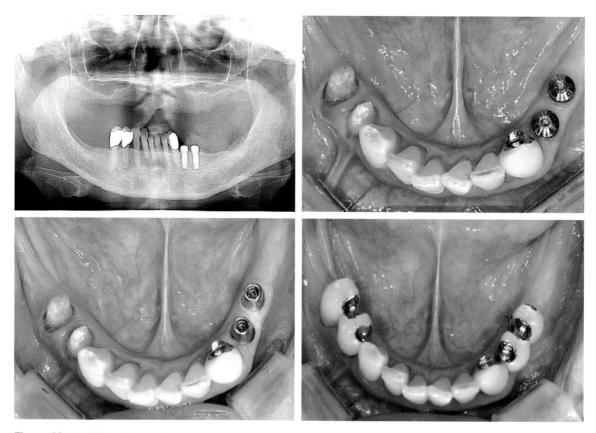

**Figure 23.** An RPD using two implant-surveyed crowns in the mandible. The symmetry between the left and right sides can be achieved by placing implants at the lower-left first and second premolar sites.

When the abutment teeth are arranged from the lower left canine to the lower right second premolar, the left edentulous area is long enough to transfer a significant amount of vertical stress on the remaining residual ridge, and the clasp placed more anterior to the fulcrum line may create rotational stress on the abutment tooth (Figure 24A). An accurate impression of the edentulous area will ensure that a more stable, well-fitting denture is fabricated. Figure 24B shows the case in which the symmetrical arrangement of the abutment teeth evenly distributes additional support. The lateral force exerted on the abutment teeth in the posterior area during mastication can also be minimized by placing the clasp posterior to the fulcrum line (compare the arrows in Figure 24).

When designed as displayed in Figure 25, the RPD can be more stable during mastication. Such an RPD design does not require bone grafting and has clasps designed to allow a slight movement of the denture, in turn reducing the harmful forces exerted on the implants. It should be noted that the RPD should have proper occlusal contact in the posterior area, and should also be relined periodically.

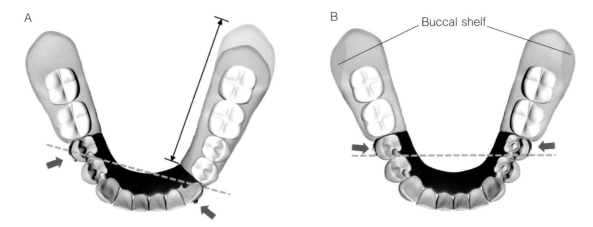

**Figure 24.** Benefits of an RPD design in which the bilateral premolars are used as abutments for the RPD. Compared to (A), (B) includes an RPA clasp that allows rotational movement about the fulcrum line. Also, the edentulous area is in the molar area, which more effectively distributes support to the abutments and the soft tissue of edentulous areas.

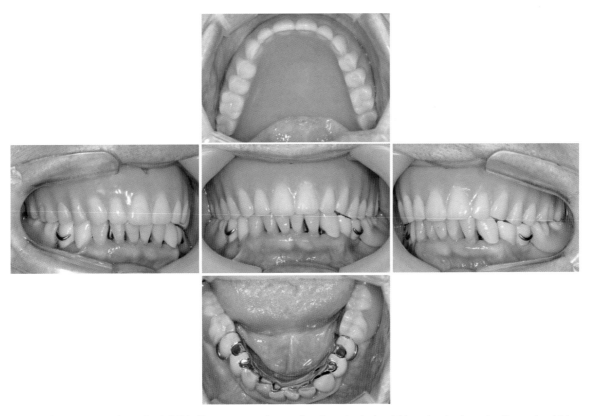

**Figure 25.** Delivery of the final RPD. Proper posterior occlusal contact should be checked, and relines should be made regularly.

**Case #2:** A 68-year old female who started wearing her maxillary and mandibular RPDs a year ago complained of an ill-fitting mandibular RPD and a fracture in a mandibular anterior tooth. The extraction of the lower left canine was necessary due to the root fracture and root caries.

As shown in Figure 26, the patient only had five (the extraction of the lower left canine was necessary) natural teeth in the mandible. The prognosis of an RPD using the five remaining mandibular anterior teeth as abutments is predicted to be worse than that of a traditional RPD using six mandibular anterior teeth as abutments. Implant placement in the posterior area was not possible given the patient's residual bone level.

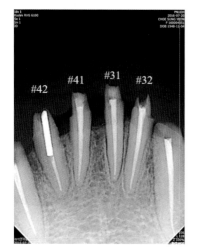 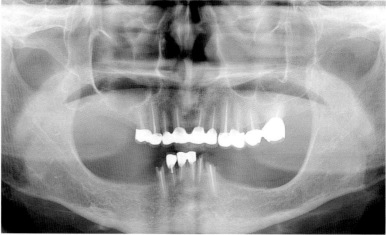

**Figure 26.** Radiograph taken during the first visit. The extraction of the lower left canine was necessary, and the rest of the mandibular anterior teeth were splinted after the restorative procedure.

As shown in Figure 27, the occlusal plane was abnormal, but the left maxillary arch displayed sound natural teeth. Recommended treatment included the fabrication of an RPD using either attachments or implant-surveyed crowns, with the implants being placed in the lower left and right first premolars.

Based on the CT scan, the treatment plan involved placing the implants at premolar sites because the opposing dentition remained intact.

A three-month healing period is necessary after the implantation. Temporary prostheses are always needed to protect the remaining anterior teeth by securing posterior support and evaluating vertical dimensions.

Gingivectomy or a crown lengthening procedure of the anterior teeth was performed to get proper ferrule. As shown in Figure 30, the anterior temporary crowns should include lingual rests for proper support,

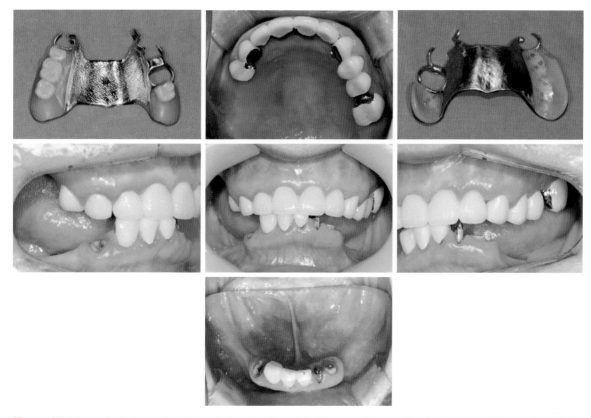

**Figure 27.** Intraoral photographs taken during the first visit. The maxillary occlusal plane was abnormal, and the remaining mandibular anterior teeth were not in a good condition.

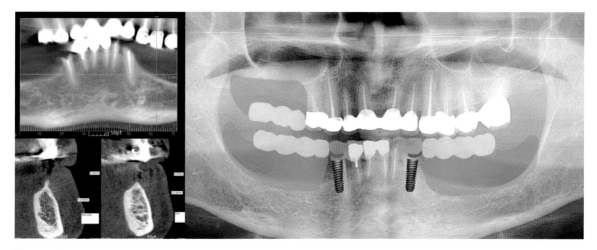

**Figure 28.** Using CT data to confirm suitability for implant placement at the lower first premolar sites.

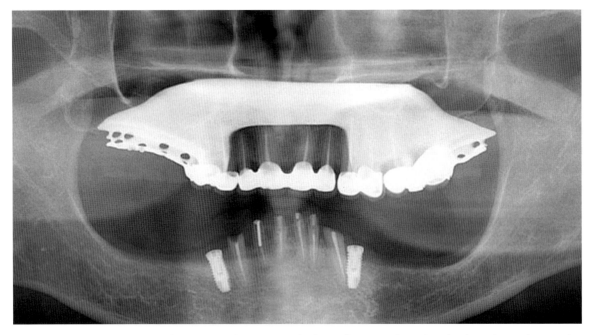

**Figure 29.** Radiographs taken after implant placement at the lower first premolars sites. Implantation and extraction were performed simultaneously.

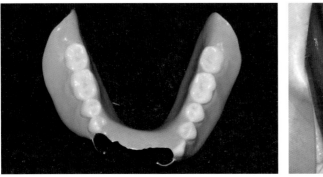 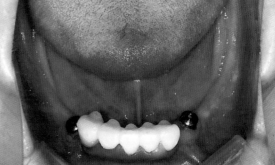

**Figure 30.** Delivery of temporary crowns and RPD after implantation.

and guiding planes must be considered. A temporary RPD must cover all the rests so that the natural dentition can provide some vertical support.

The abutments and zirconia crowns were fabricated as shown in Figures 31 and 32. Then, they were delivered as shown in Figure 33. As seen in Figure 31, a cement-retained prosthesis was chosen because of the necessity of the rest seat on the occlusal surface. In this case, the prosthesis may become detached during repeated RPD insertion or removal; to avoid such a phenomenon, the customized abutments were designed with a slight mesiodistal tilt from the path the of the RPD insertion. However, it should

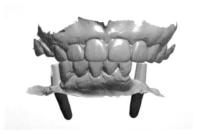 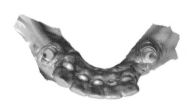 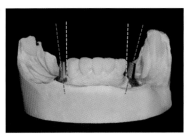

**Figure 31.** Fabrication of a customized abutments. The angulation of the implant- abutment away from the RPD path of insertion was intended. The prosthesis may become detached during RPD insertion or removal; to avoid such an occurrence, the customized abutments were designed with a slight mesiodistal tilt from the path of RPD insertion.

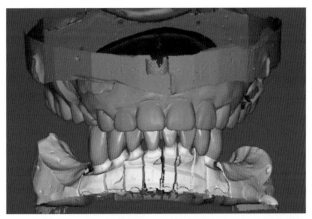

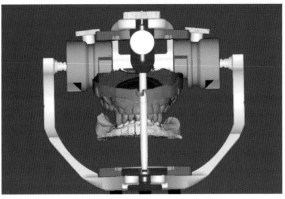 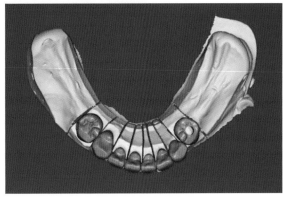

**Figure 32.** Fabrication of zirconia crowns according to the vertical dimension established with a temporary RPD. A rest seat was not formed on the lower left canine since it acted as a cantilever connected to the left implant surveyed crown. A lingual rest was designed on the rest of the anterior teeth so that the vertical force could be delivered axially. The implants and natural teeth were not splinted together.

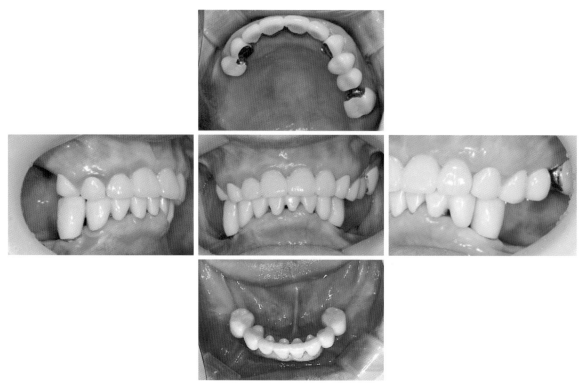

**Figure 33.** Delivery of the bridge supported by natural teeth and the implant surveyed crowns.

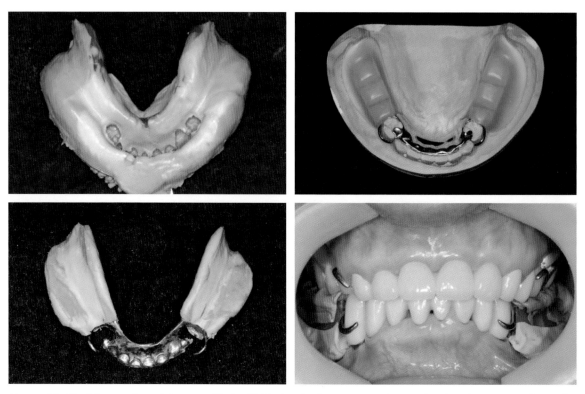

**Figure 34.** Final impression of the mandibular RPD. A selective-pressure impression is taken to transfer molar support to the edentulous area.

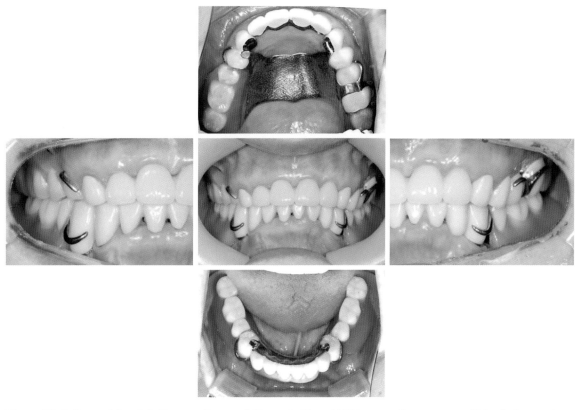

**Figure 35.** Delivery of the definitive prostheses: A Kennedy Class I RPD covers the area up until the first premolars. The occlusal contact points in the posterior teeth should be properly adjusted, and the reline performed thereafter. The patient was satisfied with the result, but ideally, the maxillary prosthesis could have been reconstructed to restore the occlusal plane.

be noted that an excessive tilt can create an ill-shaped prosthesis.

On the right side, the maxillary natural teeth occluded with the lower implant as shown in Figure 33, and the implant at the lower-left first premolar came in contact with the upper left first premolar, successfully dispersing most of the masticatory force away from the implant.

In an IARPD, the occlusal force transferred to the posterior edentulous area should be supported by the buccal shelf area using the selective-pressure impression technique as presented in Figure 34. First, an anatomic impression should be taken with a ready-made tray. Then, a custom tray can be constructed on a metal framework for the second impression. Figure 34 shows the correct technique for taking a buccal impression (see Chapter 3.3).

**In patients with an edentulous mandible, can implants be placed in the left and right canines to be used as abutments for an RPD?**

This is one of the most frequently asked questions. It is dangerous to design an RPD that incorporates two implants with individually surveyed crowns at the canines.

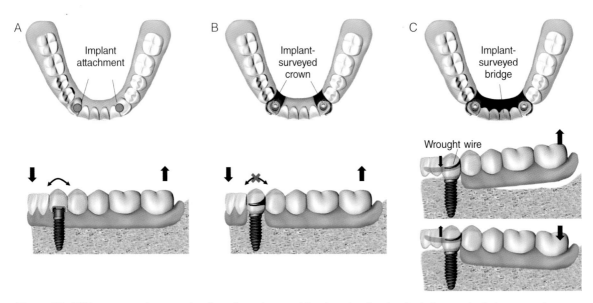

**Figure 36.** RPD movements can arise from three types of treatment using implantation on both lower canines.

Consider the three treatment plans shown in Figure 36. The treatment in Figure 36A involves the installation of attachments that allow for denture movement. If the support from the edentulous area is weak, the anterior part will be lifted when the posterior part of the denture is pushed down and *vice versa*. However, since the attachments can tolerate some degree of rotational movement, the implants will not be significantly affected by a lateral force. On the other hand, in Figure 36B, the implants are shown to act as abutments. The abutments should have guiding planes, which determine the path of insertion and can improve the stability of the RPD. Specifically, the RPD may grasp and swing the implant abutments, and a lateral force may be directly exerted onto the implants, which may be very dangerous. If such a treatment is necessary, however, the RPD must be relined frequently to ensure posterior tissue support and maintain the proper bilateral balanced occlusion. Figure 36C demonstrates the splinting of the two implants to fabricate a bridge with six anterior teeth. Compared to the second treatment plan displayed in Figure 36B, splinting the two implants will surely yield more success. Anterior tilting is blocked by the lingual rest of the anterior pontic teeth. Also, the lingual rest may also act as an indirect retainer, which helps the direct retainer to disengage from the RPD more vertically, thereby reducing the lateral rotational force. In this case, the guiding planes should be created on the distal surfaces of both canines so that the grasping and swinging of the implants can be reduced. Consider, then, the issue with lifting in the posterior region. Even though the RPI or RPA allows for denture movement, the lateral force can still affect the implants since the clasps are positioned more anteriorly than the fulcrum line. Therefore, the use of wrought wires and periodic relining are highly recommended.

> **Keypoint**
>
> When two bilaterally placed implants are used as RPD abutments in edentulous patients, the RPD is tightly bound by the abutments. This may create a seesaw (Class I lever) movement, which directs the lateral rotational force directly onto the implants. Therefore, such treatment can be very dangerous. However, it may still be adopted if the opposing dentition is a complete denture, or if the RPD can be confined by the impression and occlusal scheme. Additionally, this type of treatment will require high maintenance.

# REFERENCES

1. De Carvalho WR, Barboza EP, Caula AL. Implant-retained removable prosthesis with ball attachments in partially eden-tulous maxilla. Implant Dent. 2001;10:280-284.

2. Eom JW, Lim YJ, Kim MJ, Kwon HB. Three-dimensional finite element analysis of implant-assisted removable partial dentures. J Prosthet Dent. 2017;117:735-742.

3. Gharehchahi J, Asadzadeh N, Mirmortazavi A, Shakeri MT. Maximum dislodging forces of mandibular implant-assisted removable partial dentures: in vitro assessment. J Prosthodont. 2013;22:543-549.

4. Keltjens HM, Kayser AF, Hertel R, Battistuzzi PG. Distal extension removable partial dentures supported by implants and residual teeth: considerations and case reports. Int J Oral Maxillofac Implants. 1993;8:208-213.

5. Mijiritsky E. Implants in conjunction with removable partial dentures: a literature review. Implant Dent. 2007;16:146-154.

6. Shahmiri R, Das R, Aarts JM, Bennani V. Finite element analysis of an implant-assisted removable partial denture during bilateral loading: occlusal rests position. J Prosthet Dent. 2014;112:1126-1133.

7. Werbitt MJ, Goldberg PV. The immediate implant: bone preservation and bone regeneration. Int J Periodontics Restor-ative Dent. 1992;12:206-217.

8. Wismeijer D, Tawse-Smith A, Payne AG. Multicentre prospective evaluation of implant-assisted mandibular bilateral distal extension removable partial dentures: patient satisfaction. Clin Oral Implants Res. 2013;24:20-27.

9. Yeung S, Chee WW, Torbati A. Design concepts of a removable partial dental prosthesis with implant-supported abut-ments. J Prosthet Dent. 2014;112:99-103.

10. 10. Bae EB, Kim SJ, Choi JW, Jeon YC, Jeong CM, Yun MJ, Lee SH, Huh JB. A Clinical Retrospective Study of Distal Extension Removable Partial Denture with Implant Surveyed Bridge or Stud Type Attachment. Biomed Res Int. 2017;2017:7140870.

11. Oh YK, Bae EB, Huh JB. Retrospective clinical evaluation of implant-assisted removable partial dentures combined with implant surveyed prostheses. J Prosthet Dent. 2020 Aug 10;S0022-3913(20)30297-3. doi: 10.1016/j.prosdent.2020.04.018. Online ahead of print.

*Chapter 4-3.*

# Fabrication of IARPDs using implants with attachments

Chapter 4.1 introduced examples of clinical cases in which healing abutments or attachments were used on a small number of implants in distal extension RPDs to provide posterior support. This section will cover the factors that need to be taken into consideration when installing implants with attachments in patients who have their remaining teeth arranged in an arch, such as in a crossed occlusion.

When the remaining teeth exist unilaterally as in a crossed occlusion, the rotational axis of the RPD is formed by a line connecting the residual teeth mesiodistally, resulting in displacement to the right or left. A study by Kweon et al.(2000) suggested that if an implant is placed on the opposite side of the residual dentition, the rotation of the RPD can be prevented by diversifying the rotational axes. Such treatment can also more effectively enhance the stability and masticatory efficiency as compared to the traditional RPD treatment.

### Question

**Is it safe to install implants with solitary attachments (stud-type attachments) in the edentulous area of the patients who have unilateral teeth remaining in the maxilla?**

### Answer

Implants with solitary attachments seem to present too many complications when used in IARPDs, particularly in the maxilla. Thus, solitary attachments are applied only if sufficient stability is established by the remaining teeth in the maxilla. If the maxilla has poor bone quality, the use of IARPDs and overdentures may put the implants at risk, as the dentures may wrench the solitary attachments and impose an undesirable lateral force onto the implants.

The survival rate of implants in mandibular IARPDs (both RPD and overdentures) is relatively high. On the other hand, in the maxilla, factors such as the remaining bone volume, bone quality, implantation site, and functionality contribute to the relatively low survival rate of implants used with maxillary IARPDs. According to studies by Goodacre et al.(2003), the survival rate of implants in IARPDs is the lowest among other implant prostheses treatments, with the 5-year survival rate of implants being less than 71%. Some clinical studies comparing the survival rates of implants in the maxilla and mandible also reported a higher failure rate in the maxilla.

However, splinting the maxillary implants may help raise this survival rate. Splinting adjacent implants yields mechanical benefits, including an even distribution among the implants and enhanced cross-arch stabilization. A systematic review by Cehreli et al.(2010) reported that splinting, abutment type, and implant size do not influence the implant survival rate. However, further clinical studies are necessary to establish standard treatment guidelines for maxillary IARPDs. Earlier studies have investigated implant survival merely through main validity variable analysis and provided ambiguous descriptions of the RPD fabrication and prosthetic complications. The reason for variability in implant survival rate in maxillary IARPDs may be attributed to the foundational factors that may contribute to denture stability. Taken together, however, the survival rate of the implants in maxillary IARPDs appears to improve with carefully constructed RPDs designed to maximize the vertical force and minimize the lateral force exerted on the implants.

The 72-year old male patient shown in Figure 1 previously received three implants in the maxillary edentulous area and an IARPD from another hospital. The patient presented with pain in the posterior-most implant (upper right second premolar site) and recurring fractures in the RPD.

The patient presented with a deep bite. Furthermore, in the mandible, all of his remaining teeth were restored with porcelain-fused-to-metal (PFM) crowns after root canal treatment. In the maxilla, the first two anterior implants had locators, while the posterior-most implant did not seem to have osseointegrated properly. Also, the occlusal rests at the upper left first and second premolars were broken, and the state of the denture indicated that it had already been repaired.

The problems with his earlier treatment were as follows:

(1) The patient had a decreased vertical dimension of occlusion and demonstrated a deep bite. His masticatory force was relatively strong as the opposing dentition was composed of several natural teeth.

(2) Two of the three implants were narrow implants with a length of 8 mm. The implants were located

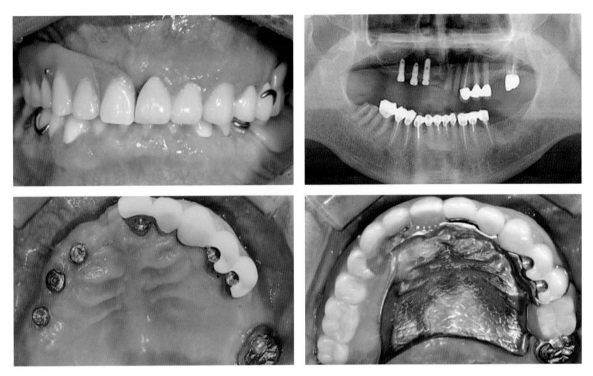

**Figure 1.** Intraoral photographs taken during the initial visit. The patient had unilaterally remaining natural teeth in the maxilla and was given an IARPD after receiving short implants in the maxillary edentulous area.

more buccally, compared to the path of insertion of the RPD guided by the restored natural teeth. Thus, the locator attachments were crushed during insertion and removal of the RPD.

(3) The fractures in the occlusal rests located on the upper first and second premolars resulted in high subsidence (tissue-ward movement) of the RPD, thereby unevenly distributing the masticatory force. Therefore, the implants on the right-hand side seem to have been overly burdened.

(4) Due to insufficient vertical space, applying the bar to splint the implants was deemed impossible. As shown in Figure 2, about 14 mm of vertical space is required for the bar(Pasciuta et al (2005)).

(5) An excessive masticatory force was loaded on to the implants instead of the edentulous alveolar ridge, resulting in recurring fractures of the RPD base.

The recommended treatment involved a full mouth rehabilitation as well as restoration to increase the occlusal vertical dimension, but the patient agreed only to a maxillary RPD due to age and cost concerns. Therefore, the finalized treatment plan was as follows:

(1) Removal of the implant in the maxillary right second premolar site which failed to osseointegrate.

(2) Enhancement of minor connectors on the maxillary left first and second premolars' occlusal rests, and the

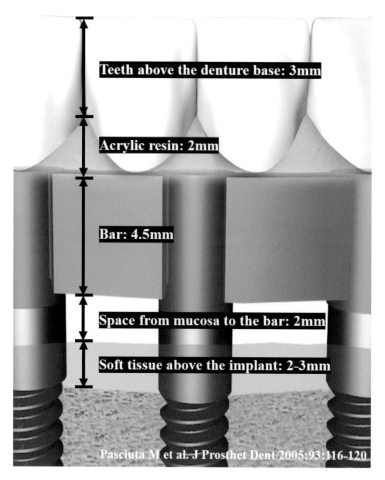

Teeth above the denture base: 3mm

Acrylic resin: 2mm

Bar: 4.5mm

Space from mucosa to the bar: 2mm

Soft tissue above the implant: 2-3mm

Pasciuta M et al. J Prosthet Dent 2005;93:116-120

**Figure 2.** The vertical space necessary for a bar application.

addition of an interdental rest between the maxillary left lateral incisor and canine to provide maximum vertical support to the natural dentition.

(3) Prosthetic modification of the guiding planes to unify the path of insertion of the RPD, and intraoral adjustment of the abutments to create sufficient thickness in the minor connectors.

(4) Fabrication of a well-fitting metal framework where the proximal plate and minor connectors should be positioned.

(5) Modification of the denture to structurally provide more support, and replacement of the base material with metal to prevent further fractures.

(6) Formation of uniform occlusal contacts between the natural and artificial teeth, and removal of the posterior occlusal contact points that were created during lateral movement.

It is critical to inform the patient about the unfavorable prognosis of the implants and the potential necessity for repair if the implants fail.

The RPD was refabricated according to the treatment plan detailed above, as shown in Figure 3. Efforts to strengthen the metal framework and to provide additional tissue support in the edentulous area to prevent the excessive offload onto the implants are shown in Figure 4. After removing the implant in the maxillary right second premolar site, locator attachment systems that allow for a limited range of movement were chosen for a more even distribution of support to the posterior edentulous region. Efforts to evenly distribute the masticatory force to each of the left and right posterior teeth were also made.

During the one year follow-up, the patient did not experience any major discomfort, but the implant was under excessive strain, as expected. This case emphasizes the need for regular check-ups and maintenance.

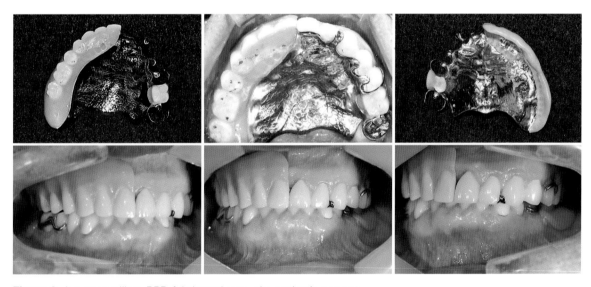

**Figure 3.** A new maxillary RPD fabricated upon the patient's request.

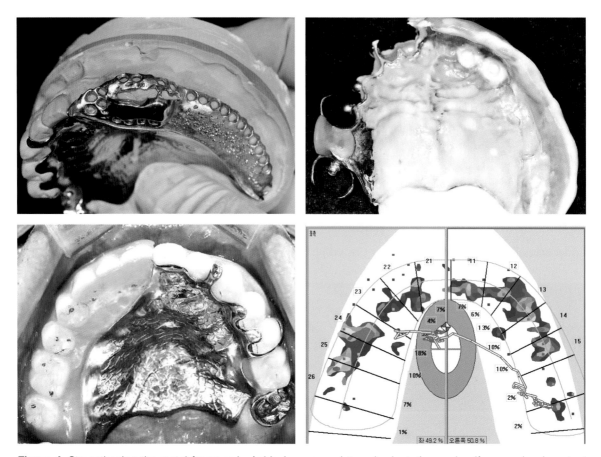

**Figure 4.** Strengthening the metal framework. Achieving proper internal adaptation and uniform occlusal contact points.

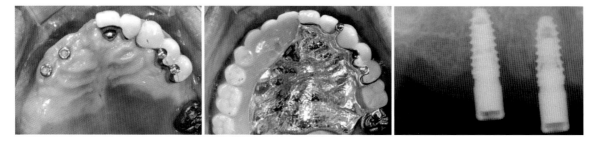

**Figure 5.** Intraoral photograph and radiograph taken during the one year follow-up. The patient presented no major discomfort, but an excessive force was transferred to the implant as expected.

> **Keypoint**
>
> Support should be evenly distributed throughout the implants, natural teeth, and edentulous tissue to act against the strong masticatory force. Sufficient stability should also be provided by the natural dentition. Furthermore, efforts to maximize support and stability of the RPD itself should always be taken.

**Question**

## Where should implants be placed in patients with a crossed occlusion?

**Answer**

It is challenging to fabricate a stable RPD for patients with a crossed occlusion. Moreover, restoring the occlusion in patients whose centric relation is lost and the occlusal plane is severely adjusted presents mechanical difficulties. Also, the reestablished occlusion may not be stable in the long term. Therefore, RPDs fabricated for crossed occlusion treatment incorporate multiple rests on the remaining abutment teeth as well as rigid type retainers, such as telescopic RPDs, for extensive support. However, if additional support is given excessively to the unilaterally remaining teeth, this may not necessarily help the survival of the abutment teeth. Therefore, the ideal treatment for patients with a crossed occlusion involves restoration of the vertical dimension and implant placement in defective areas. The implant installation should provide stability when faced with the rotational tissue-ward movements of the RPD. When the remaining abutment teeth are arranged unilaterally, the implants should be placed symmetrically on the other side, and they should occlude with opposing natural teeth.

The 66-year-old female patient shown in Figure 6 wore both maxillary and mandibular RPDs and came in experiencing pain in the mandibular edentulous area as well as discomfort resulting from inefficient mastication. It was decided not to do a reline because she had a crossed occlusion, and implants were instead placed in the lower-left canine and second premolar sites with locators to utilize the existing dentures and address the problems at hand.

The locator attachments on the lower-left canine and second premolar sites create the a design of a Kennedy Class I RPD that uses bilateral abutment prostheses.

The implant at the second premolar site paired with a locator attachment allows slight movement and creates a fulcrum line (indicated in redline in Figure 7) with the lower right second premolar, the posterior-most abutment tooth. Both the locator at the lower left canine site and the rests located more anterior to the fulcrum line (yellow arrows in Figure 7) act as indirect retainers. This allows vertical disengagement of the locator at the lower left second premolar site and the clasp at the lower right second premolar site, lifting the posterior part of the RPD.

Pushing down on the posterior part of the denture (red arrows in Figure 7) would rotate the posterior part of the RPD and cause it to subside around the fulcrum line. Here, the clasp at the lower right first premolar site may exert a lateral force on the abutment tooth via a Class I lever action. The locator attachment at the left canine site can reduce tissue-ward movement of the distal extension denture. The blue arrow indicates

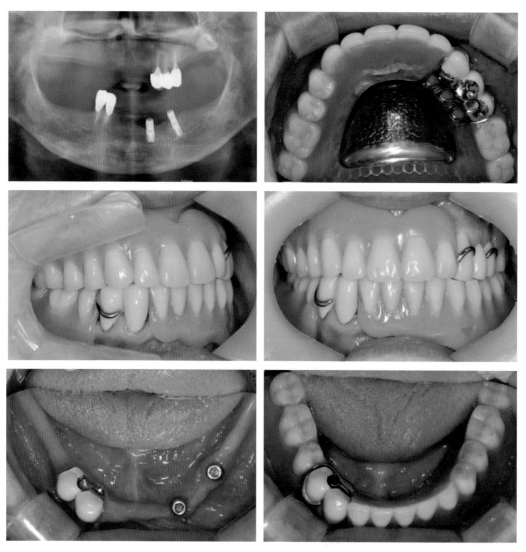

**Figure 6.** Implantation site in a patient with a crossed occlusion. Rotational movement of the RPD can be effectively reduced if designed with left-and-right symmetry and implants come in occlusal contact with opposing natural dentition.

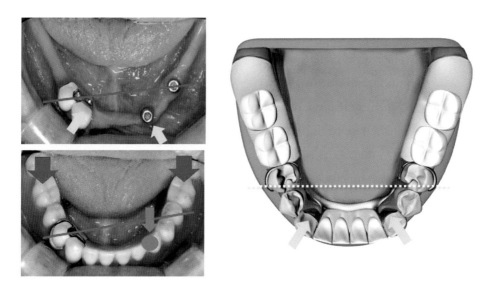

**Figure 7.** Understanding the role of two attachments. Locators enhance support and retention. The locator at the canine site also acts as an indirect retainer and offers cantilever support. For additional information, see Chapters 2.3 and 2.5.

that the additional retention offered from the locator can also reduce the subsidence of the posterior area. This illustrates the concept of cantilever support as described in Chapter 2.5.

It is important to understand that if only a healing abutment were to be used at the left canine site rather than the attachment, it would act as an indirect retainer, but would not offer cantilever support. However, cantilever support is not always advantageous. Excessive wear on the attachment in close proximity to the fulcrum line can ultimately transfer increased lateral force to the implant. Therefore, rather than simply relying on cantilever support, relines of denture base should be periodically performed to ensure the reduction of tissue-ward movements of the RPD.

### Question

**What are the factors that should be taken into consideration when choosing an appropriate attachment system for the IARPD?**

### Answer

There are several attachment systems made up of different materials. They differ in terms of resistance to wear and tear, affordance of movement, level of retention, and permitted range of implant angulation. Therefore, there is no single best attachment system. Attachment systems can be divided into three major categories: stud, bar, and magnet attachments. The selection of an appropriate attachment system depends on a multitude of factors: patient preference, retention rate, rotational movement affordance, relationship with the opposing dentition, and space available for the attachment in the RPD. Literature has shown that the choice of the attachment system does not affect the success of the implant. Thus selection should be made based on whether the mechanical properties of the attachment fit the desired needs, and whether maintenance is possible in the case at hand.

However, some principles should be adhered to when dealing with attachments in RPDs, regardless of which system is used.

---

**Keypoints**

1. When more than two implants are installed, the implants should be placed parallel to each other. Make sure that the angle of implantation falls within the permitted range of the chosen attachment system.
2. The path of insertion of the IARPD is generally decided by the arrangement of the remaining teeth. If there are only one or two remaining teeth and multiple implant attachments, the path of insertion can instead be determined by the location of the attachments. Regardless of how it is determined, however, the path of insertion of the RPD should always be parallel to, or within the permitted range of, the angle of the implants.

---

Commercially available attachment systems have various permitted ranges of the angle at which implants are installed when two or more attachments are used. Some products claim to tolerate up to 30 degrees; however, according to a studies by the author [Kim et al.(2015), Choi et al.(2017)], retention of the attachment drastically diminishes with repeated insertion and removal, even when performed within the permitted range of implant angulation. Thus, it is advantageous to install implants parallel to the path of insertion of abutment teeth when possible.

Also, two studies by Hirata et al.(2015, 2017) showed that implants may be bent and deformed even when the abutment system compensates for the angle of the implants installed for the RPD. Fayaz et al.(2015) also reported that a large amount of stress was still exerted on the implants when the path of insertion of the RPD was reflected on prostheses of inclined implants. In conclusion, implants installed parallel to each other and perpendicular to the occlusal plane yield the highest success.

A 68-year-old male patient presented with extreme discomfort from his old RPD. The maxillary prosthesis had been treated by his previous dentist while the mandibular prosthesis was fabricated 20 years ago. The patient refused a reconstruction on the mandibular RPD as he experienced no discomfort with it. Three implants were placed at the upper left second premolar, first molar, and lower left first

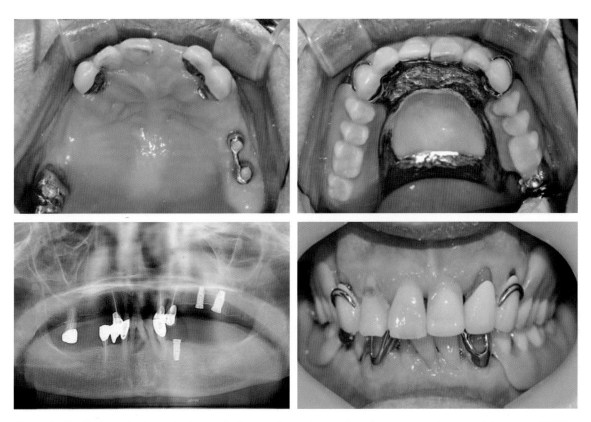

**Figure 8.** Application of a bar attachment in the maxilla and a locator attachment in the mandible on an IARPD.

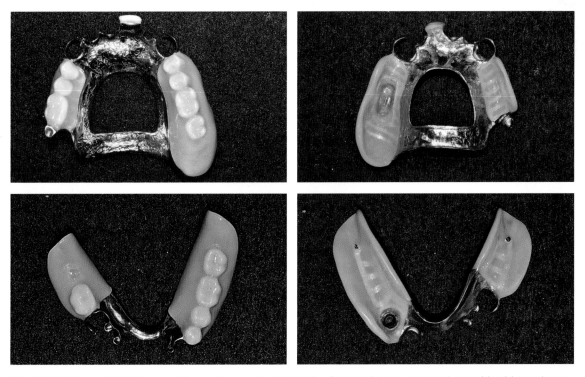

**Figure 9.** Delivery of definitive maxillary and mandibular IARPDs. Patient did not want to change his old prostheses.

premolar sites. In the maxilla, the path of insertion was determined by the anterior teeth while in the mandible, the path of insertion was determined by the existing abutment teeth, including the lingually inclined lower right lateral incisor. Therefore, implants were installed according to the path of insertion as best as physically possible (Figure 8 and 9).

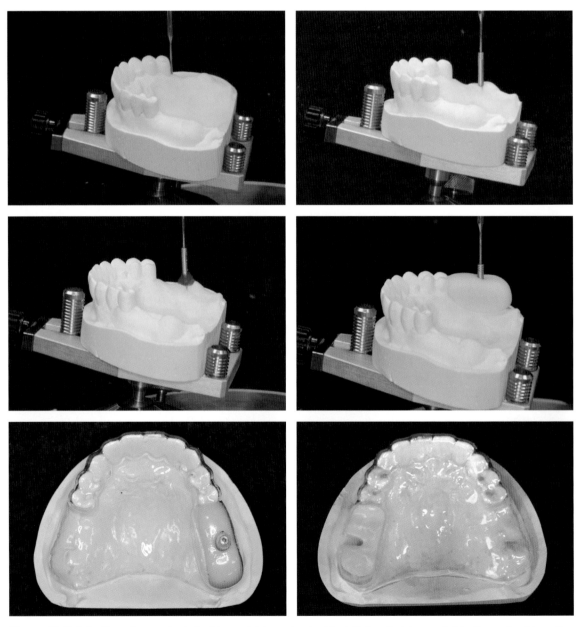

**Figure 10.** Fabrication of a surgical stent to assist in an implant installation that is parallel to the path of insertion of the RPD.

All the implants were tilted within 8 to 10 degrees of the path of insertion. Stud-type attachments appeared to be the most appropriate, but a bar-attachment was used to splint the maxillary abutment teeth, and a locator-attachment was used in the mandible. Since the prosthesis on the upper right second molar had deviated from the path of insertion, clasps were not included in the RPD design, and vertical support was provided only from the occlusal rest.

The fabrication of the maxillary and mandibular IARPDs was completed as shown in Figure 9. Wear patterns of the mandibular locator attachment were examined using a lab processing plastic sleeve after two weeks, and was then replaced with the final locator plastic sleeve. Had the angle of insertion of the implant deviated significantly from the path of insertion, implant prosthesis may have been preferable to a stud-type attachment. It should be noted, however, that the single implant prosthesis also comes with its risks.

Figure 10 demonstrates the process of surgical stent fabrication. The surgical stent can be used to place implants parallel to the path of insertion of the RPD. Once the path of insertion is chosen, the surveyor can then be moved to the expected implantation site to indicate the path of insertion with a metal rod at the implantation site. The rod can be fixed with resin, and a surgical stent can then be fabricated by vacuum forming.

> **Keypoint**
>
> Implants should be installed at an angle that falls within the permitted range offered by the selected attachment system, if not parallel to the prosthesis. This will minimize the wearing down of attachments and reduce the lateral force exerted on the implants.

It is worthwhile to examine what the attachment system enhances: retention, support, or stability.

In a case like the one shown in Figure 11, it is not possible to offer retention, support, and stability simultaneously to the RPD by a small number of attachments. The primary function of the attachment system here is to offer additional retention. Granted, the locator attachment system will provide some vertical support since its vertical movement is not significant. However, the few attachments alone should never be solely responsible for the stability of the RPD. Stability should be established by the remaining teeth as well as by the RPD design itself. The following can also be done to minimize the stress exerted on the implants and create a more even distribution: create a well-fitted metal framework, add support from the edentulous soft tissue by taking a selective pressure impression and extend the lingual flange.

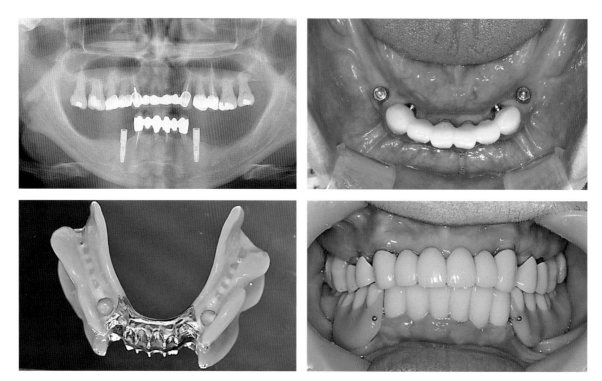

**Figure 11.** Understanding the role of the attachment system.

The primary function of the attachment system here is to offer additional retention. Granted, the locator attachment system will provide some vertical support. Stability should be established by the remaining teeth as well as by the RPD design itself.

## REFERENCES

1.  Cehreli MC, Karasoy D, Kökat AM, Akça K, Eckert S. A systematic review of marginal bone loss around implants retaining or supporting overdentures. Int J Oral Maxillofac Implants. 2010;25:266-277.

2.  Choi JW, Bae JH, Jeong CM, Huh JB. Retention and wear behaviors of two implant overdenture stud-type attachments at different implant angulations. J Prosthet Dent. 2017;117:628-635.

3.  Goodacre CJ, Bernal GB, Rungcharassaeng K, Kan JYK. Clinical complications with implant and implant prostheses. J Prosthet Dent. 2003;90:121-132.

4.  Grossmann Y, Levin L, Sadan A. A retrospective case series of implants used to restore partially edentulous patients with implantsupported removable partial dentures: 31-month mean followup results. Quintessence Int. 2008;39:665-671.

5.  Hirata K, Takahashi T, Tomita A, Gonda T, Maeda Y. Influence of Abutment Angle on Implant Strain When Supporting a Distal Extension Removable Partial Dental Prosthesis: An In Vitro Study. Int J Prosthodont. 2017;30:51-53.

6.  Hirata K, Takahashi T, Tomita A, Gonda T, Maeda Y. The influence of loading variables on implant strain when supporting distal extension removable protheses. An in vitro study. Int J Prosthodont. 2015;28:484–486.

7.  Kay KS, Kim YS, An JK. A clinical study on rehabilitation of vertical dimension in the patient with crossed occlusion. Oral Biology Res. 2001;25:127-143.

8.  Keltjens HM, Kayser AF, Hertel R, Battistuzzi PG. Distal extension removable partial dentures supported by implants and residual teeth: considerations and case reports. Int J Oral Maxillofac Implants. 1993;8:208-213.

9.  Kim SM, Choi JW, Jeon YC, Jeong CM, Yun MJ, Lee SH, Huh JB. Comparison of changes in retentive force of three stud attachments for implant overdentures. J Adv Prosthodont. 2015;7:303-311.

10. Kweon HS, Kim MJ, Moon IH. A clinical study on using Konus telescope removable partial denture in presthetic treat-ment for maxiillary and mandibular teeth cross each other. Oral Biology Res. 2000;24:201-214.

11. Mitrani R, Brudvik JS, Phillips KM. Posterior implants for distal extension removable prostheses: a retrospective study. Int J Periodontics Restorative Dent. 2003;23:353-359.

12. Mohamed GF, El Sawy AA. The role of single immediate loading implant in long class IV Kennedy mandibular partial denture. Clin Implant Dent Relat Res 2012;14:708-715.

13. Pasciuta M, Grossmann Y, Finger IM. A prosthetic solution to restoring the edentulous mandible with limited interarch space using an implant-tissue-supported overdenture: a clinical report. J Prosthet Dent. 2005;93:116-120.

14. Raghoebar GM, Meijer HJ, Slot W, Slater JJ, Vissink A. A systematic review of implant-supported overdentures in the edentulous maxilla, compared to the mandible: how many implants? Eur J Oral Implantol. 2014;7:191-201

15. Schneider AL, Kurtzman GM. Bar overdentures utilizing the Locator attachment. Gen Dent. 2001;49:210-214.

16. Stoumpis C, Kohal RJ. To splint or not to splint oral implants in the implant-supported overdenture therapy? A systematic literature review. J Oral Rehabil. 2011;38:857-869.

17. Wismeijer D, Tawse-Smith A, Payne AG. Multicentre prospective evaluation of implant-assisted mandibular bilateral distal extension removable partial dentures: patient satisfaction. Clin Oral Implants Res. 2013;24:20-27.

18. Zitzmann NU, Marinello CP. Treatment outcomes of fixed or removable implant-supported prostheses in the edentulous maxilla. Part II: clinical findings. J Prosthet Dent. 2000;83:434-442.

19. Fayaz A, Geramy A, Memari Y, Rahmani Z. Effects of Length and Inclination of Implants on Terminal Abutment Teeth and Implants in Mandibular CL1 Removable Partial Denture Assessed by Three-Dimensional Finite Element Analysis. J Dent. 2015;12:739-46.

Chapter 4-4.

# IARPDs using a combination of implant bars and attachments

Attachments used for implant-assisted dentures are divided into solitary and splint types, depending on whether implants are connected to each other or not. In the solitary type, implants are not connected to each other. This type is more readily used because maintaining hygiene is easier and technical sensitivity is lower. As previously explained in Chapter 4.3, however, successful prostheses require that implants are parallel to one another, and to the path of RPD insertion, and also that the implants are located at an appropriate distance from one another. Compared to a solitary type, a splint type attachment has higher stability, provides more support, and demands less frequent check-ups, but it requires a certain intermaxillary distance and sufficient bucco-lingual space.

### Question

**What are the advantages of using a bar in an IARPD?**

### Answer

In terms of patient satisfaction and masticatory efficiency, an implant fixed prosthesis is better than a removable prosthesis. However, if the patient has excessive vertical space due to vertical bone resorption or lingually placed implants due to buccal bone resorption, a fixed prosthesis is not effective because it cannot form the ideal tooth shape with the given conditions. It also becomes difficult for the patient to maintain a level of oral hygiene, thereby increasing the susceptibility to peri-implantitis. Also, for patients with severe bone resorption, a fixed prosthesis would not be aesthetically pleasing, as the soft tissue, such as those in the lips and cheeks, cannot provide sufficient support.

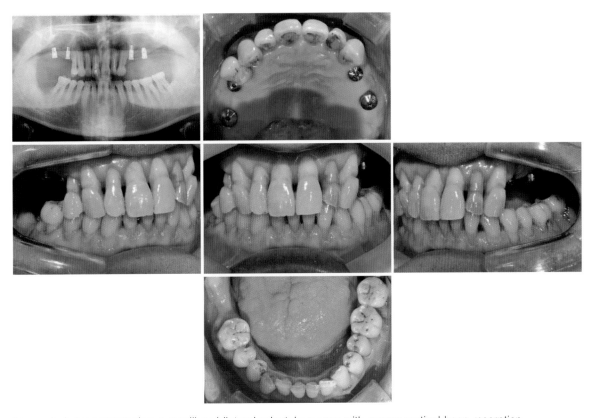

**Figure 1.** A case presenting a maxillary bilateral edentulous area with severe vertical bone resorption.

The following cases illustrate the advantages of using bars and attachments in IARPD.

Figure 1 shows the intraoral photos of a 64-year-old male with diabetes and hypertension. Maxillary molars were extracted due to generalized periodontitis, and his remaining teeth extend from the upper right first premolar to the upper left canine.

Generally, the residual teeth had the degree one mobility (only buccolingual mobility), The problems with this patient were as follows:

1) Although support was provided by a temporary denture after periodontal treatment, the residual teeth had shown slight mobility due to alveolar bone resorption around the teeth.

2) Even though the amount of vertical bone resorption on the maxillary molar area was quite severe, surgeries such as vertical bone augmentation were not an option because of his systemic diseases.

3) Though additional implants could have replaced the extracted teeth, due to poor prognosis of the residual teeth, the patient asked for prostheses that were easy to maintain and repair for economic reasons.

4) If treated with a fixed prosthesis, the edentulous molar area would likely experience vertical bone resorption, resulting in an elongated crown and a lack of tissue support. This would not only cause food impaction but also make cleaning difficult. Additionally, the fixed prosthesis would not support the buccal cheek area, bringing about aesthetic concerns.

5) Since the lower opposing natural teeth were sound, balancing the inter-occluding force between the maxilla and the mandible was necessary.

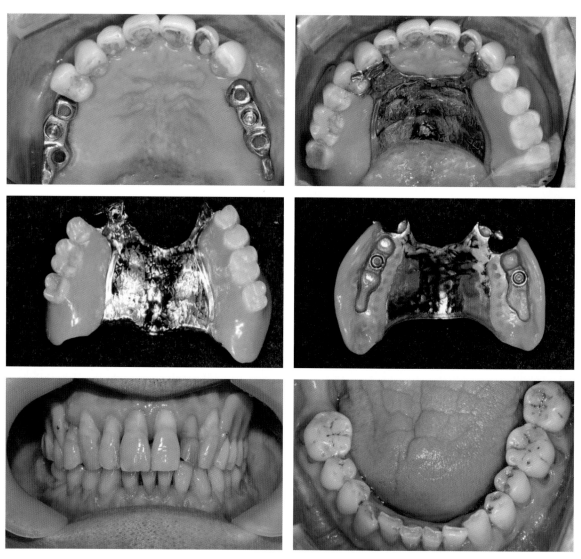

**Figure 2.** Post-treatment photographs of the IARPD that used bars and dedicated attachments.

Two implants were placed on each maxillary molar area where a bone graft was not needed. As shown in Figure 2, customized abutments were manufactured on the implant installation site, and both a milled bar and locator attachments were used. Then, the abutments and the attachments were bonded together using resin cement. The fit between the bar and the metal framework of the RPD is particularly important in this type of structure. However, the bar attachment presents three major disadvantages: the fabrication process is complicated, the production costs are high, and the quality is extremely variable and dependent upon the individual technician's skills. Also, it becomes more difficult to repair once the initial friction is gone. On the other hand, when using a milled bar and a attachment, the adaptability is not as important. This is because there is additional retention provided by the attachment, and additional stability and support provided by the lateral and upper wall of the bar. As shown in Figure 3, support, and stability are all provided by the bar alone, and the rests distribute vertical support to the residual teeth. The two locators on the bars provided enough retention, so the circumferential clasps were not needed on the natural teeth.

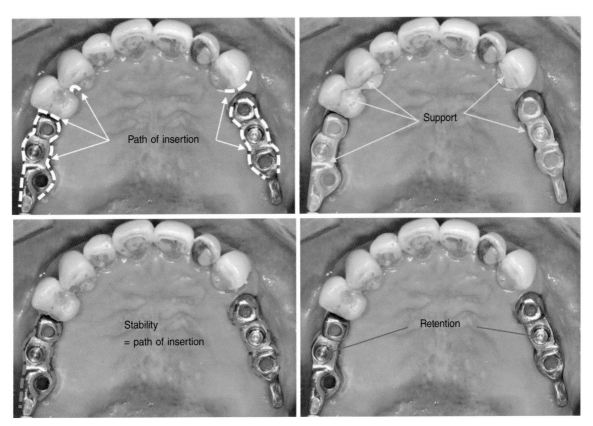

**Figure 3.** Post-treatment photographs of the IARPD, which incorporated both bars and locators.

The parts of an IARPD that offer retention, support, and stability are labeled separately in Figure 3. All RPD components must be arranged parallel to the path of insertion. The left and right bar pathways should be parallel to the path of insertion of the RPD as well as that of the residual teeth. When the residual teeth consist of maxillary incisors, a surveyor should be used to establish a parallelism between the path of insertion of distal and proximal teeth as well as the minor connector that is connected to a rest. This not only allows the easy insertion of RPD but also dramatically improves its stability. The yellow areas in Figure 3 indicate the RPD support areas. The maxillary implants are rigidly connected, and the superior surface of the bar is parallel to the patient's occlusal plane. This provides support for the molar area, but also adds additional support to the residual teeth. Even the teeth with mobility can benefit from the enhanced vertical support provided by the additional occlusal rests.

The locators in the bar provide retention to the RPD. A circumferential clasp is not applied here because any kind of lateral force would put the mobile teeth at great risk given the extent of the modifications already made on the teeth. Using locators offers the advantage of increasing the lifespan of the retention apparatus given that the male and female attachment parts can be regularly replaced as needed. It is also easy to ensure the parallelism of the path of insertion of the locator by a bar with threads for the locator screw. In the case of the patient shown in Figure 3, the plastic sleeve of the locator was replaced after two years of using the IARPD. Though there are concerns about possible abrasions on the locator abutments after long term use, as the bar have internal threads for the locator screw, they can be easily replaced as needed.

The suggested treatments addressing the aforementioned problems were as follows:

1) After periodontal treatment, although support was provided on the molar area with a temporary denture, the residual teeth had shown mobility due to the alveolar bone resorption around the teeth.

   : Occlusal rests were created on the residual teeth, and the path of insertion of various RPD components and minor connectors were all made uniform to enhance the support and stability of the denture. The attachment apparatus, which consisted of bars and locators, also minimized the lateral force exerted on the residual teeth.

2) Even though the amount of vertical bone resorption on the maxillary molar area was high, vertical bone augmentation was not an option because of the patients systemic disease.

   : Since the patient was not treated with implant fixed prostheses, a simple implant surgery could be performed on areas that did not require a bone graft.

3) The prognosis of the residual teeth was not favorable and therefore it was explained that additional implants would be placed when the teeth were extracted. For economic reasons, however, the patient

wanted a prosthesis that was easy to maintain and could be repaired easily.

: The patient was given an RPD with a bar attachment. This would make hygiene maintenance and dental repairs easier, even with the additional loss of incisors.

4) If treated with a fixed prosthesis, the edentulous molar area would experience vertical bone resorption leading to a lengthened crown and a lack of tissue support. This would not only cause food impaction but also make cleaning difficult. Also, the fixed prosthesis would not support the buccal cheek area, causing an unaesthetic facial contour.

: Fabricating an IARPD seemed ideal, given its easy maintenance and ability to disguise the loss of soft tissue with the denture base.

5) Since the opposing natural teeth were sound, it was necessary to balance the inter-occluding forces between the maxillary and the mandibular arch.

: Abrasions and fractures are unavoidable, but the metal framework was strengthened during the manufacturing process to prevent such damage. However, if there are abrasions to the artificial teeth, the occlusion should be monitored to ensure that the occlusal force transferred to the residual incisors is not excessive, given the reduction in support offered from the molar regions. Should the wear become severe, however, the occlusal surface of the artificial teeth can be restored with a more sturdy material such as metal. In this patient's case, the splinted implants provided support strong enough to endure the occluding force from the mandibular teeth.

### Question

**When fabricating an IARPD that uses a milled bar and an attachment, in which parts of the IARPD are parallelism important?**

### Answer

As previously explained, three parts should be parallel to one another: the lateral surface of the bar, the path of insertion of the attachment, and the distal and proximal surfaces of the residual teeth. Additionally, the path of insertion of the minor connectors should also be made parallel if they are located between the teeth.

The patient shown in Figure 4 had been previously treated with implant fixed prostheses at another clinic but had some failed implants and four remained implants. A milled bar was used and three locators were installed, so an additional clasp was considered unnecessary. In a bilateral distal extension RPD, the path

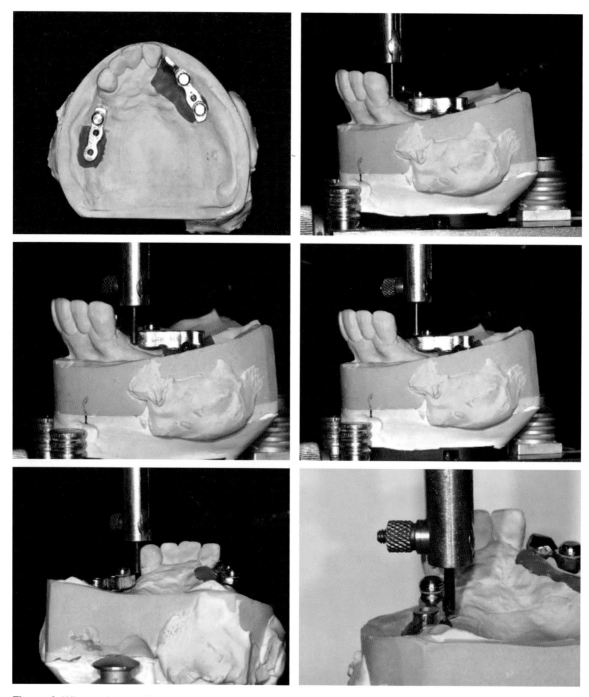

**Figure 4.** When using a milled bar and an attachment for an RPD, all components of the bar should be parallel to the path of insertion of the RPD. The lateral surface of the bar, the path of insertion of the attachment, and the distal and proximal surfaces of the residual teeth should be parallel to prevent attachment wear and exertion of harmful lateral forces.

of insertion is determined by the distal surface of the most posterior residual teeth, where the proximal plate is typically located. If the surface of these teeth are not uniform, they can be slightly trimmed. Then, the newly formed path of insertion should be made parallel to the lateral surface of the milled bar and the path of insertion of the attachment. As mentioned in Chapter 2.4, denture stability can be enhanced when the path of insertion and removal is different from the path of dislodgement.

---

**Keypoint**

If the patient had been treated with an RPD with circumferential claps on the maxillary residual teeth, it would have been difficult to make appropriate undercuts for the clasps. Also, considering the undercut of the maxillary incisors, it would become more complicated to match the lateral surface of the milled bar to the path of insertion of the RPD. If the paths of insertion of the milled bar and the maxillary incisor were different, harmful lateral forces would have been exerted on the residual teeth upon every insertion and removal of the RPD.

---

**Question**

**Is a locator necessary when using a milled bar? If different attachment systems were used, would it pose any problems?**

**Answer**

Other types of attachments could also be used. Regardless of the specific attachment system used, the role is the same, namely to provide retention.

Figures 5A and 5B emphasize how the gold clip allows rotational movements and in turn enhances retention. It allows for the tissue-ward movement of the distal extension denture. Figures 5C and 5D are displays of four implants installed and connected with bars and clips. The bar attachments are rigid and the three clips are placed in each bar, preventing any denture movement. Figures 5E and 5F demonstrate how using a milled bar and a magnet attachment will prevent any movement. Additional retention is provided by the magnet in this case. Figures 5G and 5H show the milled bar case with an ADD-TOC® attachment (PNUADD Co., Ltd., Busan, Korea) that was developed by the author. The concept of the ADD-TOC® attachment is similar to the locator, but the diameter is smaller than the locator and the components of the attachment can last without severe abrasion or deformation for a long time.

When using a bar with various attachment systems, even if the attachment itself allows movement,

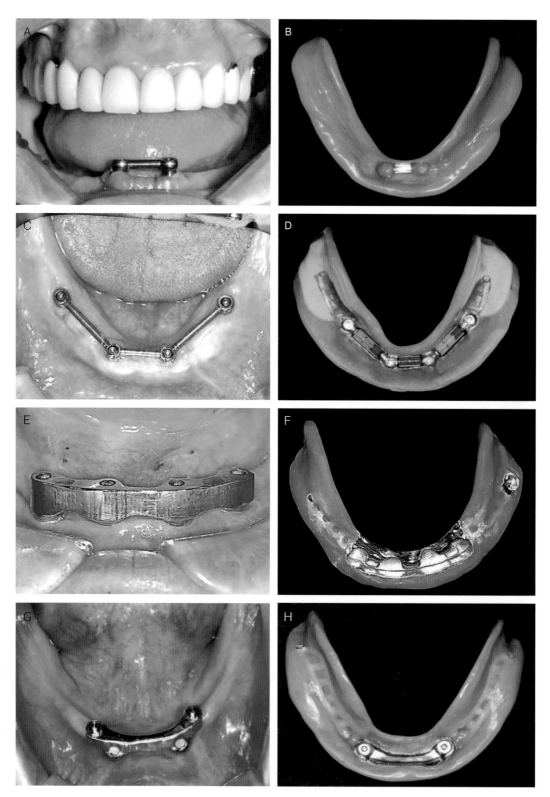

**Figure 5.** Different methods of applying a bar and attachments.

if the multiple attachments are placed in different positions on the bar, the attachment system as a whole becomes rigid and prohibits any kind of movement from the denture. In this rigid system, the attachment may also provide support and stability. The use of a milled bar is preferred when retention, support, and stability are all demanded from the bar. Take, for example, Figure 5. In Figures 5A and 5B, two implants are connected by a bar. Retention is enhanced by the gold clip which allows for rotational movements. In this case, the clip not only provides retention, but also allows the rotational and tissue-ward movements of the distal extension denture. The anterior implants also provide some support, and the clip and the bar provide some additional stability. Here, the tissue-ward movement of the denture is allowed. This is called a resilient type of bar attachment. In Figures 5C and 5D, four implants are connected by bars and clips. With only one clip, the bar attachment allows for rotational movements. However, when three clips are all placed without being parallel, the bar attachment becomes rigid and does not allow for any movement by the denture. In this case, though the denture may have been manufactured to provide sufficient support and stability, the three clips provide most of the support, retention, and stability. It should be noted, however, that if the opposing teeth are natural teeth or the occluding force is too strong, the clip may form abrasions or undergo deformations, and the denture itself may even break. Figures 5E and 5F showcase the use of a milled bar and a magnet attachment. In this case, movement is not allowed, and additional retention is provided by the magnet. The better the milled bar fits with the metal apparatus of the RPD, the stronger the retention of the denture by frictional forces and the greater the stability provided by the lateral wall. For IARPDs that require a bar, the use of a milled bar is recommended so that not only are support and stability guaranteed regardless of the attachment type selected, but also potential abrasions to the attachment can be reduced.

The following case is an example of an IARPD with a milled bar and Hader bar attachment.

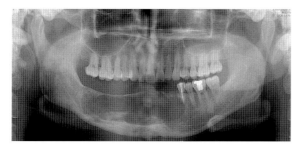 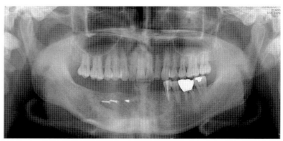

**Figure 6.** The initial panoramic image taken of a 43-year-old male patient. Multilocular radiolucency was seen in the right mandibular area, and it was later diagnosed with ameloblastoma.

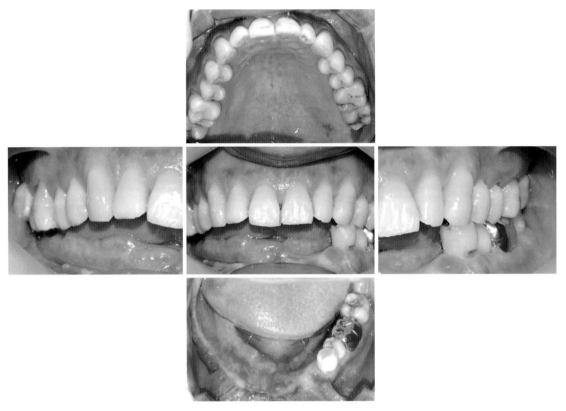

**Figure 7.** Intra-oral pictures taken after surgery.

In a Hader bar attachment, the bar and sleeve are made of plastic. This bar can be burnt out and is castable with any type of metal, and is therefore frequently selected for use. However, in this case, the Hader bar was fabricated with a CAD/CAM system, not by traditional casting methods. Figures 8-12 show the entire treatment process.

This case displays a Kennedy Class II patient, who has lost all of his mandibular right teeth and left incisors. His mandibular residual teeth were sound. Opposing teeth consisted of natural dentition. Even after a bone graft conducted by surgery, alveolar bone loss was still significant.

Impressions were taken with silicone and a master cast was made. The master cast was then scanned with a 3Shape's D700 scanner and designed using a specialized software. Labioversion of implants made it difficult to fabricate the prosthesis as a single unit. After a customized abutment was designed, taking into consideration factors such as the angle of implantation, the abutment was manufactured with titanium. The silicone index was used to evaluate the 3-dimensional space of the bar. In this case,

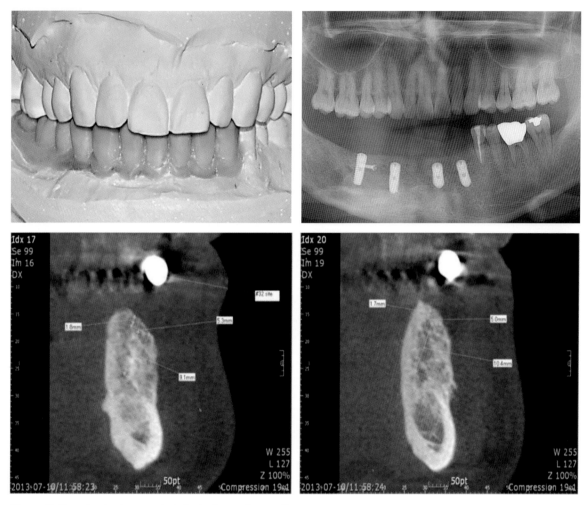

**Figure 8.** Four implants were installed after a diagnostic wax-up.

all movement of the RPD was prohibited. Because the bar and clips should provide all the support, stability, and retention, the CAD/CAM system was used to maximize accuracy.

The customized abutment and milled bar were checked intraorally, and bonded with resin cement. The installed implants were internally connected, but fortunately, the abutments, which were connected to the bars, were removable. For the fabrication of the metal framework, the milled bar was scanned, and the metal framework was designed using a software program. Here, retention was obtained from the clip, as well as from the sidewalls of the milled bar. Comparing Figure 11 with Figures 5C and 5D, it is evident that the sidewalls on the underside of the Hader bar help to maximize the stability of the denture. The designed metal framework was fabricated by milling. The framework was then fixed with impression material, and the clip was connected by a self-polymerizing resin.

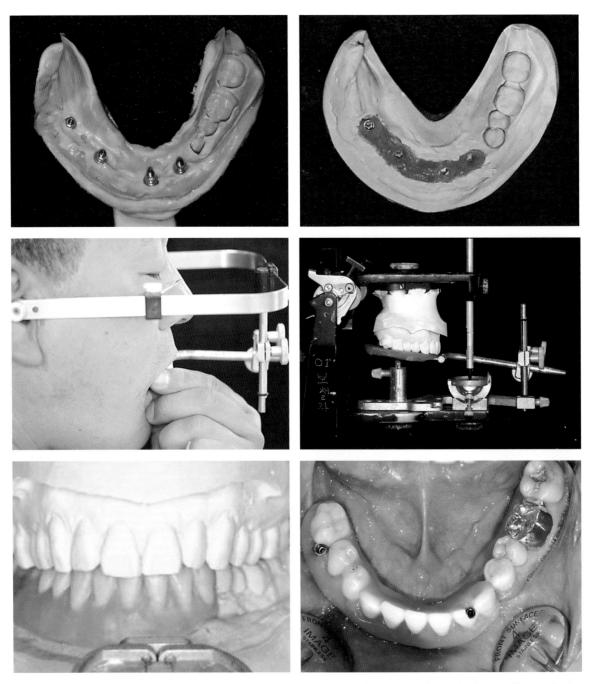

**Figure 9.** Try in of a diagnostic wax denture after a facebow transfer was performed, the maxillomandibular relationship was recorded, and the artificial teeth were appropriately arranged. When making a wax denture, a temporary abutment helps the denture to seat accurately.

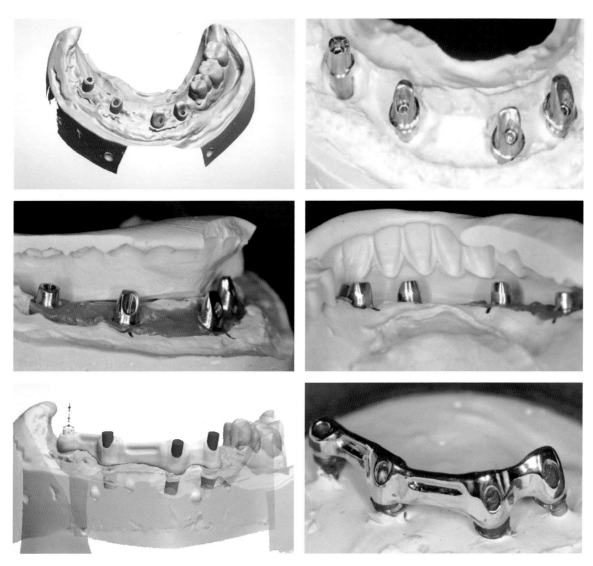

**Figure 10.** The fabrication of a customized titanium abutment. The silicone index was created to evaluate the available space for a bar using the diagnostic wax denture.

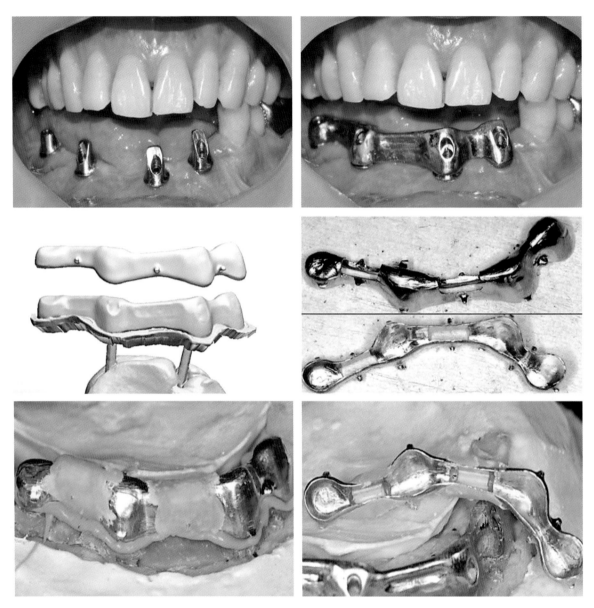

**Figure 11.** Fabrication of the metal framework to be placed inside the denture base.

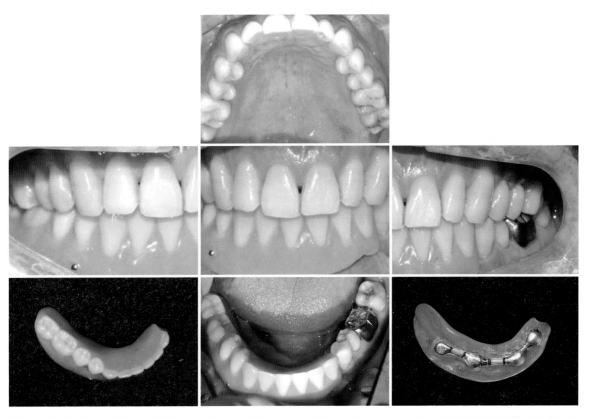

**Figure 12.** Delivery of the definitive prostheses. Although only two clips were used, retention was sufficient due to the friction from the sidewalls of the bar. A Hader bar and a milled bar were applied together. The sidewalls of the milled bar provided enough stability, and the upper surface of the bar granted enough support, making a rigid RPD that allowed no movement. Unlike the denture shown in Figures 5C and 5D, where retention, support, and stability were all obtained from the plastic clips and bar itself, this type of denture has a longer lifespan and greater patient satisfaction. Since the denture was considered to be a rigid IARPD sufficiently supported by implants, the occlusal adjustment was made in the same way as for natural dentition; a group function and mutually protected occlusion was established.

### Question

In an edentulous patient with severe alveolar bone resorption, the locators tend to wear out too quickly when two implants are placed anteriorly. This may be due to a failure to establish parallelism with the implant installations. Is it better to use a milled bar to splint the two implants and then place two locators in parallel? Will the locators be more resistant to wear in this way?

### Answer

There may be several reasons why locators tend to wear out when using stud-type attachments with

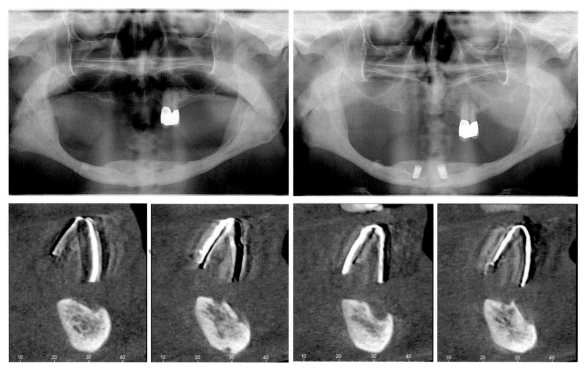

**Figure 13.** Radiographs taken at the initial visit and after implant placement.

two anteriorly placed implants in the mandible. As the question suggests, it could happen because the angles at which the implants were placed were not the same. It can also occur because the dentures do not sufficiently cover the edentulous soft tissue, leading to a lack of support and thus resulting in unwanted denture movement. Using a Hader or Dolder bar with two implants, whether a stud or bar type, will result in denture movement. However, a milled bar, as shown in Figures 5E and F, will not allow any movement because it will create a friction-retained denture. This is a rigid type attachment. When using this type of rigid attachment on the implants, especially if the milled bar is in full contact with the metal framework, one should take into consideration the fact that all denture movements will be prevented, potentially leading to a significant exertion of an external force on the implants.

The following case describes a patient with an overdenture with a milled bar and two implants.

Figure 13 are radiographs of a 76-year-old male with a maxillary RPD fracture. The patient wanted reconstruction of a mandibular complete denture. The existing dentures were made 10 years ago and the maxillary RPD fracture occurred two months ago. The patient did not receive regular maintenance checks, and there was no unusual medical history. The abutments on the upper left canine and first premolar did not have any secondary caries, mobility, or unusual radiographical features. The maxillary residual ridge showed substantial horizontal and vertical bone resorption, while the lower jaw showed severe horizontal and vertical bone resorption. After evaluating with a diagnostic wax-up, the vertical space of the anterior teeth and premolars were determined to be greater than 12 mm. As such, the traditional maxillary RPD and mandibular complete denture could be manufactured. In the mandible, however, the patient experienced strong discomfort because of severe alveolar bone resorption, so an implant overdenture was planned as part of treatment.

Because the maxillary denture was fractured and the mandibular denture did not fit properly, temporary dentures were used until the completion of implant osseointegration. Implants were placed at the lower right lateral incisor and left lateral incisor sites using a surgical stent (Figure 14). Because of the poor bone quality of the patient, parallel placement of the two implants was impossible, and even the distance between the two implants was closer than ideal (about 6 mm).

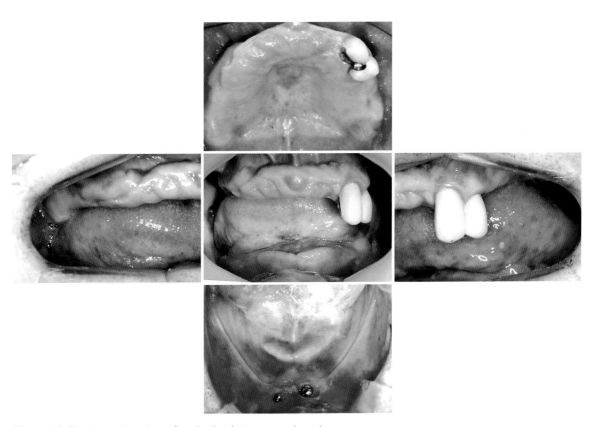

**Figure 14.** Photographs taken after the implants were placed.

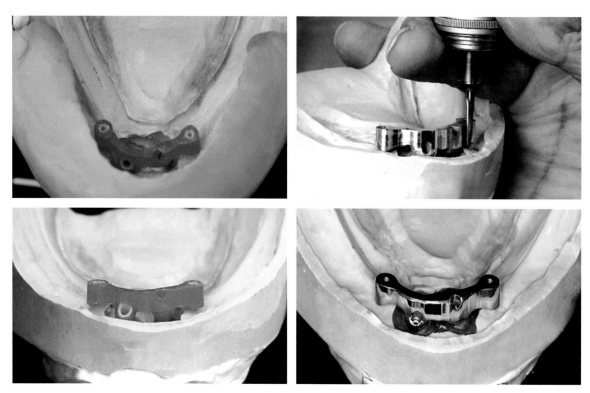

**Figure 15.** After making a milled bar pattern using pattern resin, a vertical and horizontal spatial evaluation between the bar and the denture was performed using a silicone index. The pattern resin was cast to produce milled bars. Because there were only two implants, instead of using a typical milled bar, an unique milled bar with free space on the lateral and lingual surface was designed to allow for some denture movement.

Because the implants could not be placed in parallel, as this would result in a solitary type overdenture with a poor prognosis, a splint type overdenture was planned. Pattern resin was used to fabricate a milled bar pattern, then the index was used to evaluate the vertical and horizontal spaces. After confirming the space, the milled bar was fabricated (Figure 15). The close proximity of the two implants also meant that applying a clip would be difficult.

On the distally extended milled bar, a locator bar attachment (Locator, Zest Anchors) was installed with a torque of 30 N/cm to enhance retention and stability (Figure 16).

The metal framework of the maxillary RPD was checked in the oral cavity for fit and the presence of other errors. Then, the maxillary and mandibular wax dentures were made to evaluate the artificial teeth arrangement, labial support, occlusion, and the fit of the milled bar and the metal framework (Figure 17).

After a fit check, the definitive dentures were fabricated after final processing, laboratory remounting, occlusal adjustments, and finishing and polishing (Figure 18). Then, the dentures were successfully delivered to the patient. The patient has visited the hospital for regular checkups for the last three and half years,

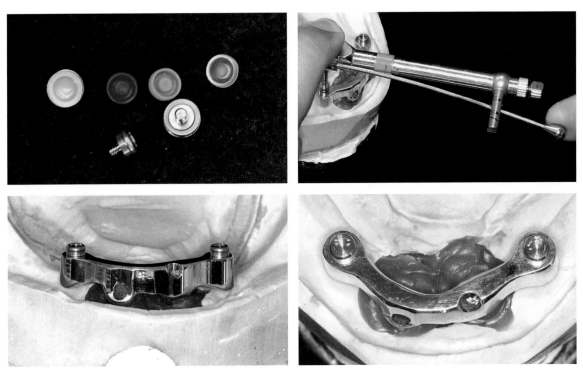

**Figure 16.** A locator was connected with 30 N/cm torque on both cantilevered sections to increase the retention of the denture.

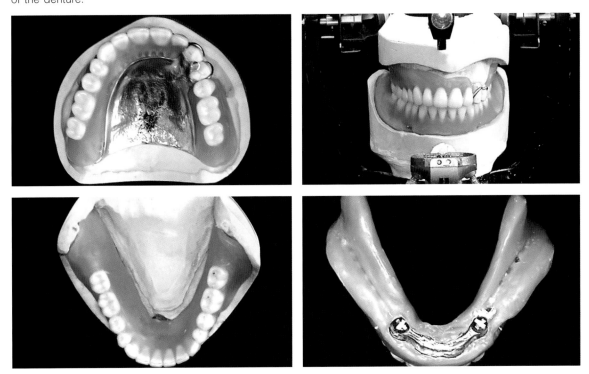

**Figure 17.** The upper and lower wax dentures were fabricated to evaluate the arrangement of the artificial teeth in the oral cavity. Lip support, occlusion, and the fit of the milled bars and metal framework were also evaluated. A bilateral balanced occlusion was established for the dentures.

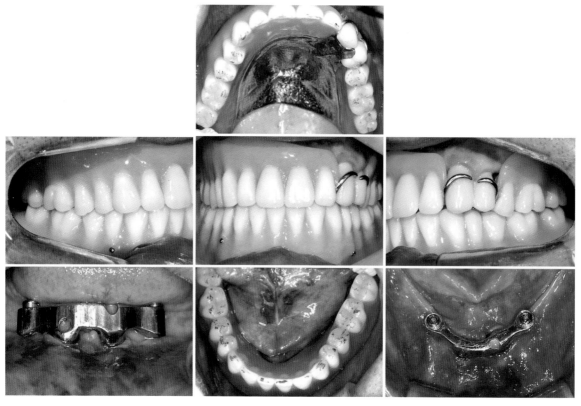

**Figure 18.** After fit checking, the definitive denture processing, laboratory remounting, occlusal adjustment, and polishing were completed. In order to minimize the denture movement, an accurate internal fit of the mandibular denture and bilateral balanced occlusion, which stabilizes the occlusion, were made.

and the dentures have been well maintained, resulting in high patient satisfaction.

Through the researches (Choi et al. 2017, 2018), seems to be parallelism of the implants is the key to a successful treatment when using a solitary type attachment. When the angular difference between implants is more than 40°, the locator attachment system shows a drastic decrease in retention. To compensate for this angular difference, angled attachments can be used. However, some studies have shown that the angled attachments make the locator vulnerable to vertical loading and that the retention is lower than when the locators were attached parallel to each other. In this case, because of severe bone resorption of the mandible, it was difficult to place more than two implants, let alone install the two implants parallel to each other. Although a bone graft could have been performed to increase the bone volume, the patient did not want to undergo aggressive surgery. Therefore, an overdenture using a bar attachment, which is less affected by implant angulation was designed instead.

Trakas et al.(2006) suggested that an implant-supported overdenture requires four or more implants while an implant-tissue supported overdenture only requires two implants to allow denture movement, with support coming from the implants and the posterior edentulous area.

According to the study by Krennmair et al.(2008), it is recommended to create a bar type overdenture with four or more implants in patients with an ovoid dental arch, like in the case presented earlier. However, since more than two implants could not be placed in this patient due to the bone condition, a milled bar that extends distally over the two implants was used. Though there was the possibility that an excessive cantilever force would be transferred to the implants, the maxillary denture was close to being a complete denture and a bilateral balanced occlusion was established to minimize denture movement. A milled bar typically does not allow denture movement in the posterior edentulous region due to its rigid and parallel-sided walls. Also, it can exert a great lateral or cantilever force on the implants, eventually leading to their failure. To avoid such a problem, a round or oval-shaped bar can be used. However, in this case, severe bone resorption resulted in deeply placed implants. Therefore, to help the patient remove and insert the RPD with greater ease, a milled bar and a guiding plane for denture insertion were made. Besides, the rear sidewall of the milled bar provided additional relief, and denture movements in the posterior edentulous region were allowed as a result. Moreover, the denture was sufficiently extended to enhance support coming from the posterior edentulous tissue. By doing all of this, as mentioned above, the rotational force exerted on the anterior implants was minimized. Furthermore, any lost retention was regained with the change of locators.

> **Keypoint**
>
> The suggested treatment for this case may seem problematic at first glance. However, if the harmful forces exerted upon the implant abutments are minimized, this type of treatment may be even more effective than using stud-type attachments.

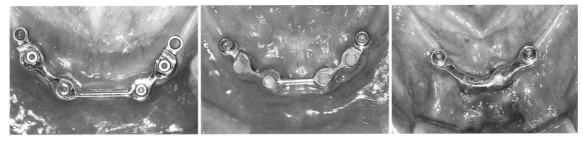

**Figure 19.** A case in which using a bar with attachments that induce tissue support permitted tissue ward movement. The first case used a clip in the anterior and an ERA attachment on the posterior cantilever. This allowed a posterior tissue-ward movement and has been widely used in the past.

Providing relief on the metal framework that comes in contact with the bar, as shown in Figure 19, can allow for the tissue-ward movements of the denture even with only two or four implants. At this point, the permitted range of movement is important to consider.

Take, for example, Figure 20. In the anterior, a Hader bar with clip attachments is positioned. Let's say that the locator attachments installed in the posterior of the bar can move about 0.2 mm vertically. Now, imagine pressing down the posterior area of the denture. The denture base would display a tissue-ward rotation about the clip attachments. To allow for such rotational movement, there must be a relief given to the lingual side of the bar. If the sidewalls of the bar come in close contact with the metal framework, such movements will not be allowed. Additionally, if the rotation goes beyond the locator's permitted range, the front clips and locators may fall out, as shown in Figure 20. However, if the clips

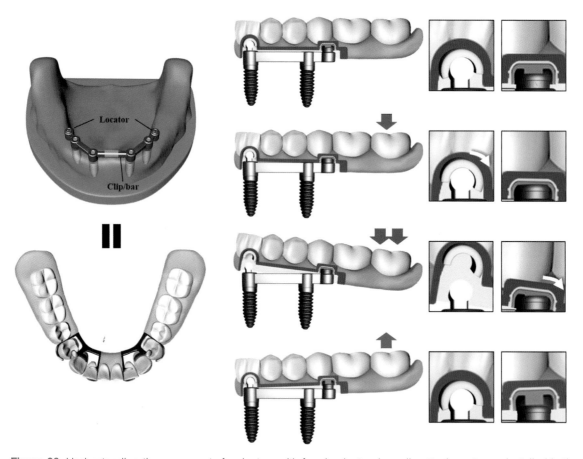

**Figure 20.** Understanding the movement of a denture with four implants when clip attachments are installed in the anterior, and locator attachments are placed in the posterior region. Such movements can be achieved when a proper amount of relief is given to the rear sidewall of the bar.

have sufficiently strong retention, they can stabilize against such rotational movement. In this case, the clip provides cantilever support, as mentioned in Chapter 2.5. The four implants are connected by a bar, so this cantilever support will not be overly harmful to the abutments. However, if there is a movement beyond the limits of the available cantilever support (retention by the clip), the denture will rotate with the locator on its center, causing the attachments to get worn down. Therefore, when using this kind of bar overdenture, regular relines of the denture base are necessary.

Now imagine the movement when the posterior part of the denture is lifted up (e.g. the movement that occurs when chewing on sticky food with the posterior artificial teeth). In order to resist dislodgement of the denture, the locators need to exert a vertical force. Here, the clips serve as indirect retainers when pushed down, and generate a vertical force on the locators, allowing them to work as direct retainers and induce vertical disengagement of the denture.

In other words, a rigid wall is created in front of the axis of rotation, which becomes an indirect retainer and increases the effectiveness of the attachment (direct retainer) (see Chapter 2.2 and 2.3).

> **Keypoint**
>
> As shown in Figure 20, an RPD that uses bars and attachments with four implants positioned anteriorly is similar to a typical Kennedy Class I RPD which should have an indirect retainer and a stress breaker type direct retainer that allows denture movement under function.

What factors should be taken into consideration when using a milled bar and a locator on two implants, as shown in Figure 21? Though this structure may appear unstable, it can still be viable if appropriate precautions are taken. As shown in Figure 20, the attachment that serves as a direct retainer is located posterior to the bar, which offers indirect retention to the anterior bar, and helps the locators to disengage vertically. Keep in mind that relief must be given to the lingual side of the metal framework to allow bar movement. Also, the bar must be sufficiently angled on the buccal side. If normal two-degree milling is done, the buccal side of the bar will disturb the tissue-ward rotation of the denture. Thus, the bar should be more tapered on the buccal side. Also, the cantilever distal to the bar cannot be overly extended. It just needs to be long enough to place the locators.

The denture movement in Figure 21 is similar to the denture movement in patients with a Kennedy Class I RPD with six remaining anterior teeth. If periodic denture base relining is not carried out, the attachment may become distorted, get worn out, or even fall out. Besides, this design can exert a lateral rotational force to the implant, so regular maintenance check-ups are essential after delivery.

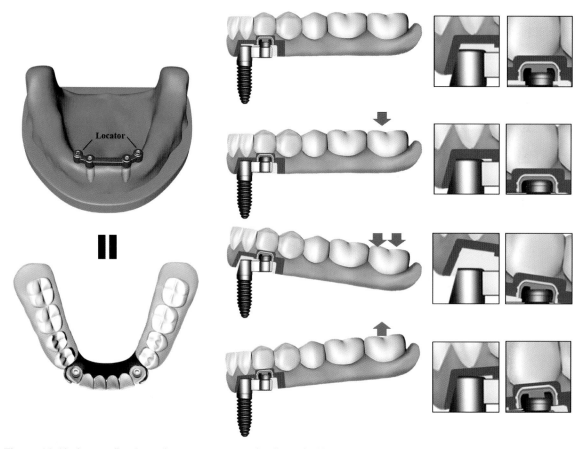

**Figure 21.** Understanding how denture movement is allowed with two implants installed in the anterior area using a bar and two locators.

However, when the implants are intentionally tilted, and the distance between the anterior and posterior implants is large, as shown in Figure 22, a bar that supports the posterior area can be designed without considering the previously mentioned movements. In this case, a rigid-type overdenture that does not permit any denture movement can be fabricated. This establishes close contact between the bar and the metal framework. If the maxilla has only a few teeth remaining or if it is completely edentulous, then this type of treatment with four implants in the mandible may be appropriate.

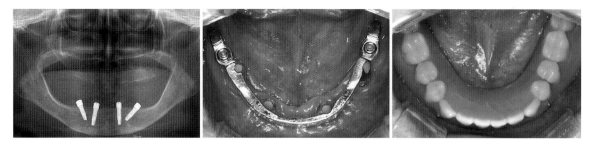

**Figure 22.** An overdenture with 4 implants that do not allow any denture movement.

# REFERENCES

1. Chan MF, Närhi TO, de Baat C, Kalk W. Treatment of the atrophic edentulous maxilla with implant supported overden-tures: A review of the literature. Int J Prosthodont. 1998;11:7-15.

2. ELsyad MA, Shaheen NH, Ashmawy TM. Long-term clinical and prosthetic outcomes of soft liner and clip attachments for bar/implant overdentures: a randomised controlled clinical trial. Journal of Oral Rehabilitation. 2017;44:472-480.

3. Gulizio MP, Agar JR, Kelly JR, Taylor TD. Effect of implant angulation upon retention of overdenture attachmetns. J Prosthodont. 2005;24:6-22.

4. Han DH, Kim SK, Kim YH. Textbook of Oral & Maxillofacial Implantology. Vol. I Basic Principles and Techniques. Daehan Publishing Co., 2004;257-59.

5. Jemt T, Book K, Lindén B, Urde G. Failures and complications in 92 consecutively inserted overdentures supported by Brånemark implants in severely resorbed edentulous maxillae: a study from prosthetic treatment to first annual check-up. Int J Oral Maxillofac Implants. 1992;7:162-167.

6. Krennmair G, Krainhöfner M, Piehslinger E. The influence of bar design (round versus milled bar) on prosthodontic main-tenance of mandibular overdentures supported by 4 implants: a 5-year prospective study. Int J Prosthodont. 2008;21:514-520.

7. Trakas T, Michalakis K, Kang K, Hirayama H. Attachment systems for implant-retained overdentures : a literature review. Implant Dent. 2006;15:24-34.

8. Zarb G A, Mericske-Stern R. Clinical protocol for treatment with implant-supported overdentures. Prosthodontic Treat-ment for Edentulous Patients: Complete Dentures and Implant-Supported Prosthesis. 12th ed. Philadelphia. 2004;498-509.

9. Choi JW, Bae JH, Jeong CM, Huh JB. Retention and wear behaviors of two implant overdenture stud-type attachments at different implant angulations. J Prosthet Dent. 2017;117:628-635.

10. Choi JW, Yun BH, Jeong CM, Huh JB. Retentive Properties of Two Stud Attachments with Polyetherketoneketone or Nylon Insert in Mandibular Implant Overdentures. Int J Oral Maxillofac Implants. 2018;33:1079-1088.

*Chapter 4-5.*

# Application of attachment systems on implants in patients with complete edentulism

This section will cover the precautions that should be taken when making an overdenture retained by two implants and stud-type attachments. In this case, a fulcrum line that allows rotational movement will be formed, similar to the one in an RPD. Though it may seem easier to make a denture that relies on two implants because of enhanced stability, retention, and support, this is not always the case. In a complete denture, the denture itself does not have a specific rotational axis. However, when using two implants, an axis of rotation is formed, and if the denture has design issues, an external force would be transferred to the implants or attachments. Therefore, extra precautions should be taken when fabricating these overdentures.

### Question

**A patient presented with pain in the mandibular edentulous residual ridge. He had been using his maxillary and mandibular overdentures for a year and he had got the plastic sleeves of his locators changed every one month. What could have possibly caused these problems?**

### Answer

The visible problems as seen in Figure 1 are as follows:

(1) The locators installed on the two implants in both the maxilla and mandible created a clear fulcrum line.

(2) Both dentures seemed to be ill-fitted.

(3) Removing the locators essentially removed all retention, indicating that there was no denture seal.

(4) The posterior part of the mandibular denture was not extended to the retromolar pad, and the short lingual denture base resulted in reduced stability of the denture. Furthermore, the inner surface of the denture had many visible areas in which adjustments had been made.

Rather than dislodging, the dentures displayed seesaw movements around the fulcrum line created by the implant attachments. When the patient opened his mouth, the maxillary denture distal to the implants fell off, and a large tissue-ward movement of the denture was observed during mastication in the mandible.

In short, the dentures were continuously experiencing a seesaw movement.

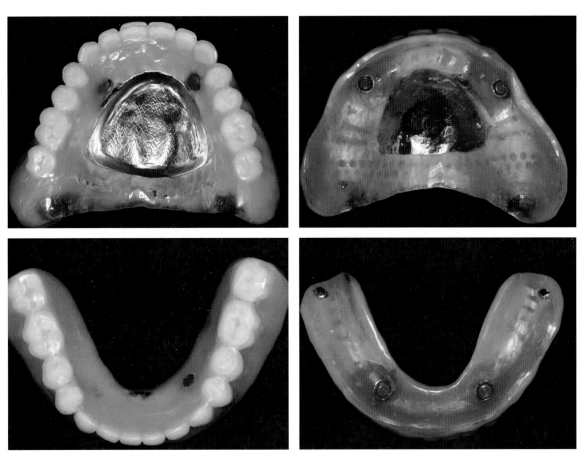

**Figure 1.** Overdentures not properly made on both sides of the maxilla and mandible. The patient experienced pain in the edentulous residual ridge of the mandible. The plastic sleeve of the locator was frequently changed because of repeated wear.

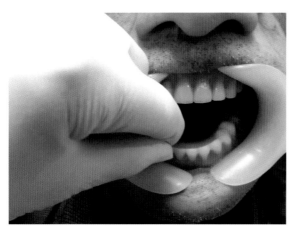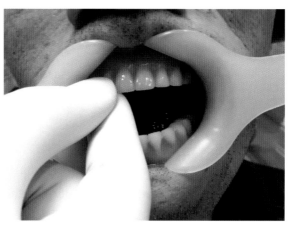

**Figure 2.** When the anterior teeth of the dentures were held and shaken by the fingers, the dentures displayed significant seesaw movement around the fulcrum line connecting the two implant attachments.

Important considerations in fabricating an overdenture relying on two implants are as follows:

(1) First, the necessity of implants should be thoroughly evaluated. The two implants in the maxilla seemed unnecessary, as a denture with sufficient retention could have been fabricated given the patient's healthy edentulous ridge. Implants should only be added to enhance retention, should the denture alone be insufficient. It is important to obtain strong support and stability from the palate and residual ridge by creating a denture with a perfect fit. Seesaw movements transfer a significant external force to the attachments, leading to poor prognoses of the implants placed in the maxilla.

(2) In the mandible, making an overdenture relying on two implants with attachments has become the normalized treatment method. An overdenture may be advantageous because it can be challenging to obtain proper retention of the mandibular denture. The implant attachments must be placed more anteriorly to decrease the likelihood of anterior rotational movement, given their added retention. A selective pressure impression technique should be used to obtain sufficient posterior support and limit the denture's posterior rotational movement. Also sufficient extension of the denture is necessary to ensure the denture's stability. Periodic relines are mandatory, and a bilateral balanced occlusion should be established to further enhance stability.

Using two implants with stud-type attachments allows rotational movements about the axis of rotation, and this is likely to cause many problems. A denture should be fabricated in a way such that it offers sufficient retention, support, and stability. Additional retention should be provided when necessary. This type of treatment is difficult and demands a lot of post-care, including frequent relinings and occlusal adjustments.

**Question**

**When many implants are installed, they can take on a multitude of roles. The patient shown in Figure 3 had five implants placed in the mandible and experienced continuous pain and abrasion of the attachments. What could be the cause?**

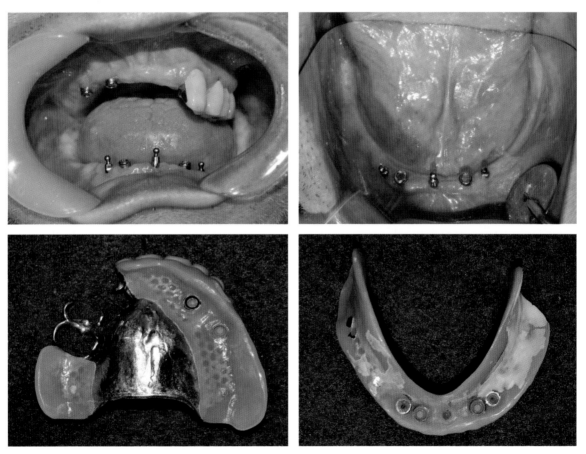

**Figure 3.** An IARPD relying on two implants in the maxilla and an overdenture relying on five implant attachments in the mandible.

## Answer

According to the patient's statement, the implants were placed in both the maxilla and mandible approximately 10 months ago, and the IARPD in the maxilla and overdenture in the mandible were used for three months and seven months, respectively. The patient was comfortable with his IARPD for the maxilla and never had to get the plastic sleeve of the locator changed. However, he experienced great discomfort with his mandibular denture. He initially had three narrow-implants (one-body implants with ball attachments), but abrasion to the attachments occurred very quickly, so he had to visit the dental office once or twice a month. His dentures were constantly adjusted to relieve the pain. However, because he exhibited a series of problems, the dentist had inserted two more implants with locator attachments. The patient felt comfortable using his mandibular denture for the first week, but the discomfort soon returned.

There are several reasons why these problems were not seen in the maxilla.

(1) There were four sound abutment natural teeth on the left side of the maxilla, and sufficient stability was provided by an embrasure clasp.

(2) The abutment teeth offered a clear path of insertion for the RPD, and the path exactly corresponded to the angle of implantation.

(3) The edentulous region in the maxilla along with a major connector with palatal coverage provided sufficient support and stability.

There were several reasons why there were multiple problems in the mandible. These are listed below.

(1) The first three narrow-implants were placed in a row. This formed only one axis of rotation even with three implants.

(2) Pain in the posterior edentulous region is indicative of severe tissue-ward movements about the axis of rotation formed by the implants. Repeated adjustments to the denture relieved the pain momentarily, but likely increased tissue-ward movements. There was no support provided by the denture base. In other words, there was no consideration given to support and stability in the denture.

(3) The additional two implants were placed in line with the existing axis of rotation. At first, the locator attachments would have prevented the movement of the denture, but repetitive rotational movements and abrasions of the locator would eventually increase the lever movements of the denture, resulting in pain in the edentulous region.

What then would be the ideal approach to treatment? As shown in Figure 4, if the two additional implants were placed in the posterior region to extend the A-P spread (space between the anterior and

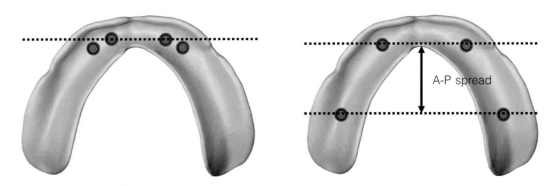

**Figure 4.** Variations of implant placement. Consideration of the space between the anterior and posterior implants (A-P spread) is important to regulate denture movement.

posterior implants), rotational movements could have been decreased. Moreover, the support provided by the denture base is less important because the posterior implants would have offered additional support.

However, insufficient bone volume may have made this difficult. If so, a reline of the denture is recommended over additional implant placement. Then, rapid abrasions to the attachments can be prevented by decreasing the rotational movements of the denture. Additionally, instead of shaving down the denture, extending it (particularly in the buccal shelf, retromolar pad, and lingual flange of denture base) and improving its fit would have caused fewer abrasions to the attachments as well as less inconvenience for the patient.

### Question

**A patient with four narrow implants and an overdenture presented with abrasions to the male part of one-body implant, and even after the o-ring attachment was replaced, retention could not be obtained. Why did the abrasion occur and how should the patient be treated?**

### Answer

Narrow implants have recently become popular in the treatment of patients with insufficient bone volume because they are more economical. It is often paired with four implants with o-ring attachments to obtain sufficient retention.

It appears that patient satisfaction is high when ball-type attachments are paired with the four implants.

However, having four implants placed in a row without proper relining can result in abrasions of the male part of the attachment.

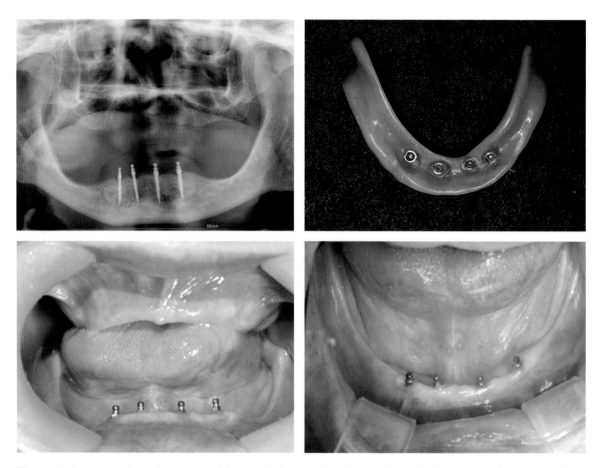

**Figure 5.** A panoramic radiograph and intraoral photographs of a patient with four narrow implants and an overdenture whose retention could not be reobtained even after a replacement of the o-ring.

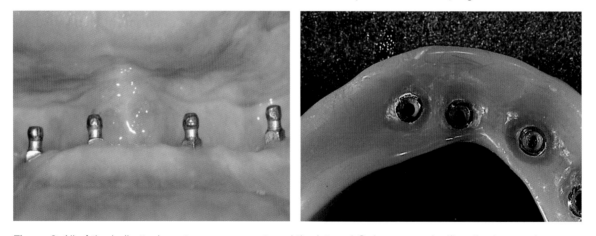

**Figure 6.** All of the ball attachments were worn out, and the internal O-rings were significantly damaged.

Figure 5 illustrates the case of a patient who had an overdenture with four narrow implants, and after two years of experiencing no discomfort, visited a dental clinic with complaints of constant pain and decreasing retention. As such, the o-ring was replaced, but the denture would still continuously dislodge.

Why did these problems occur?

(1) Narrow-implants were placed in a row.

(2) Only one axis of rotation was formed as a result of implant placement, and distal tissue-ward rotational movements of the denture occurred due to residual bone loss.

(3) As shown in Figure 5, there is little support provided by the posterior region due to an insufficiently extended denture base and the absence of a periodic relining procedure.

(4) Continuous adjustments to the internal surface of the denture base caused more rotational movements and symptoms of combination syndrome, such as maxillary anterior bone resorption, began to manifest.

---

**Keypoint**

Implants that are placed in a row make one axis of rotation regardless of the number of implants. In order to minimize the chance of abrasions, the denture itself should provide sufficient support and stability, and to minimize the rotational movement of the denture, regular relines and occlusal adjustments should be made. It is important to note that simply increasing the number of implants will not reduce denture movement.

---

It is instead recommended to add a bar attachment rather than remove or replace the implants, as shown in Figure 7.

First, the ball attachment is modified so that it can act as an abutment, and then create a bar attachment, as shown in Figure 7, by casting a Hader bar with non-precious alloys. The fabricated bar attachment is placed over the implants by using resin cement. These one-body type implants do not need the abutment to be attached like in two-piece implants. The denture should be made to provide sufficient support and stability by itself (Figure 8). Figure 7 displays the sufficiently extended border of the denture and a selective pressure impression of the buccal shelf region. Typically, only one clip attachment is used to allow for denture movement, but in this case, two clips were used because of several reasons: the bar attachment was almost entirely straight, the maxilla had a complete denture, the state of the mandibular denture was relatively good, and the denture was to be relined every six months. Two years have now

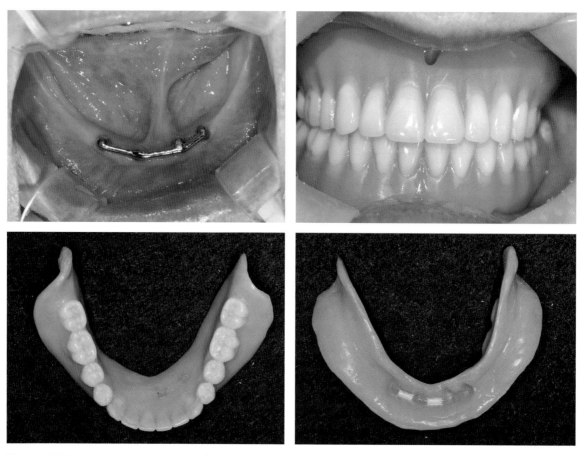

**Figure 7.** Fabrication of a new denture by changing ball attachments to bar attachments using the Hader bars from Figure 5.

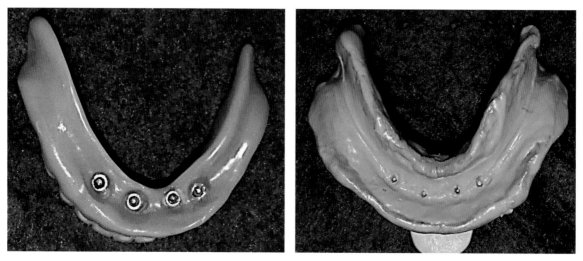

**Figure 8.** Comparison between the old denture (left) and the definitive impression taken via a selective pressure impression technique (right). The buccal shelf area was recorded extensively on the impression.

passed with consistent six month relines being performed, without the need for the replacement of a clip, and the patient expressed no discomfort.

**In an overdenture relying on two implants with stud type attachments, how can the longevity of the attachments be extended?**

The goal should be to fabricate an overdenture that can last at least a year, regardless of the types of attachments used.

In attempting to do so, four major factors should always be considered:

(1) Two implants should be placed in parallel to reduce the likelihood of abrasions to the attachments during insertion and removal of the denture.

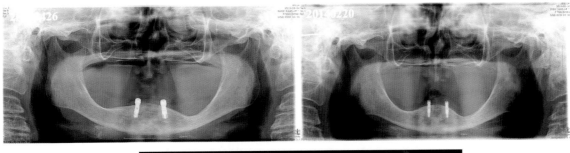

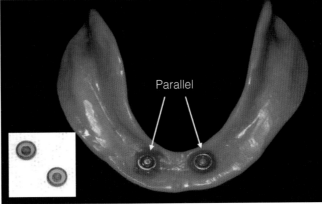

**Figure 9.** A mandibular overdenture that barely displays any abrasions to the attachments even after two years of usage.

(2) The denture should be fabricated first, and used by the patient for a few months before the implant attachments are installed. The patient should feel no discomfort with the denture (the exception is less retention).

(3) The implants should be placed in the lateral incisor region rather than in the canine or premolar region.

(4) Biannual check ups should be performed, relining the denture as necessary.

As shown in Figure 9, no abrasions of attachments were found, even after two years. Should all the four aforementioned recommendations be taken into consideration, the attachment can typically be used for longer than a year.

Dentures should be designed under the impression that no implants are to be used, so that the denture itself provides adequate support and stability. Should additional stability be needed, a bilateral balanced occlusion can be established. As shown in Figure 10, implantation in the lateral incisor site can contribute to the stability of the denture and reduce the denture's lever movements around implant attachments.

According to Figure 11, if the implant is located further in the anterior part of the jaw, the axis of rotation will be formed closer to the lower incisor teeth, decreasing the efficacy of the first class lever (i.e. when pressing the anterior teeth on the center of the rotational axis, more pressure would be needed for posterior teeth to be lifted) and minimizing the rotational movements (see Chapters 2 and 3).

Figure 12A displays a case in which the implant is placed in the anterior part of the jaw and Figure 12B displays a case in which the implant is placed in the premolar area. Imagine that there is severe movement resulting from an ill-fitting denture. According to Figure 12B, when occluding with the anterior teeth, tissue-ward movements towards the anterior region and lifting of the posterior region will occur around the rotational axis of the implant attachments. In contrast, if the posterior teeth are pressed, lifting of the anterior region occurs around the rotational axis of the implant attachments. Can these attachments last for a long time? Imagine now that the anterior region in Figure 12A is pressed down. The posterior region would not be lifted easily because of the vertical support provided by the implant placed in the anterior region (or the rotational axis and point of force are very close). In other words, an efficient inhibition of the Class I lever has been formed. In contrast, if the posterior region were to be pressed, even though the denture is assumed to be ill-fitting, because the axis of rotation and the point of force are distant from each other, the anterior region would not be lifted as much as in Figure 12B.

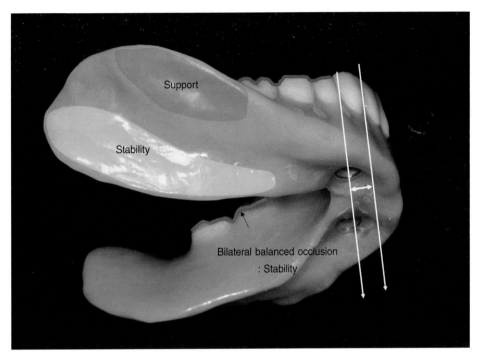

Figure 10. The denture itself should provide sufficient support and stability.

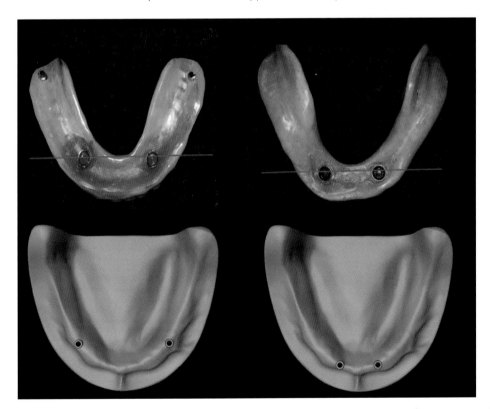

Figure 11. The difference of the fulcrum line according to the implant location. If the implant is located further in the anterior part of the jaw, the axis of rotation will be formed closer to lower incisor teeth, decreasing the efficacy of the first class lever.

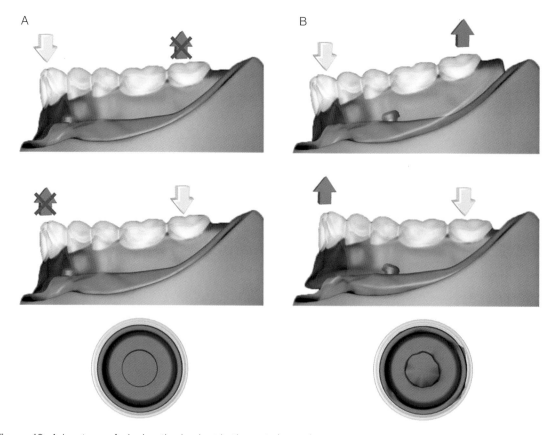

**Figure 12.** Advantage of placing the implant in the anterior region.

**Keypoint**

Many attempts have been made to minimize denture movement by placing implants in the lateral incisors instead of in the canines or premolars. However, this may not always be the perfect solution. The chosen implantation site should be able to effectively control the Class I lever actions. Additionally, regardless of the site of implants, periodic relines and occlusal adjustments can ensure the success of the treatment. Recent studies have shown that placing one implant in the center of the anterior region for an overdenture has yielded great success. This success can be attributed to the fact that the denture itself provides sufficient support and stability, and the attachments provide the necessary retention (as displayed in Figure 12).

# REFERENCES

1.  Alqutaibi AY, Kaddah AF, Farouk M. Randomized study on the effect of single-implant versus two-implant retained over-dentures on implant loss and muscle activity: a 12-month follow-up report. Int J Oral Maxillofac Surg. 2017;46:789-797.

2.  Chaves CA, Souza RF, Cunha TR, Vecchia MP, Ribeiro AB, Bruniera JF, Silva-Sousa YT. Preliminary In Vitro Study on O-Ring Wear in Mini-Implant-Retained Overdentures. Int J Prosthodont. 2016;29:357-359.

3.  Damghani S, Masri R, Driscoll CF, Romberg E. The effect of number and distribution of unsplinted maxillary implants on the load transfer in implant-retained maxillary overdentures: an in vitro study. J Prosthet Dent. 2012;107:358-365.

4.  Elsyad MA, Mohamed SS, Shawky AF. Posterior Mandibular Ridge Resorption Associated with Different Retentive Systems for Overdentures: A 7-Year Retrospective Preliminary Study. Int J Prosthodont. 2017;30:260–265.

5.  Jawad S, Barclay C, Whittaker W, Tickle M, Walsh T. A pilot randomised controlled trial evaluating mini and conventional implant retained dentures on the function and quality of life of patients with an edentulous mandible. BMC Oral Health. 2017;17:53.

6.  Scherer MD, McGlumphy EA, Seghi RR, Campagni WV. Comparison of retention and stability of two implant-retained overdentures based on implant location. J Prosthet Dent. 2014;112:515-521.

7.  Scherer MD, McGlumphy EA, Seghi RR, Campagni WV. Comparison of retention and stability of implant-retained over-dentures based upon implant number and distribution. Int J Oral Maxillofac Implants. 2013;28:1619-1628.

8.  Scherer MD. Overdenture Implants. A Simplified and Contemporary Approach to Planning and Placement. Dent Today. 2015;34:54-56.

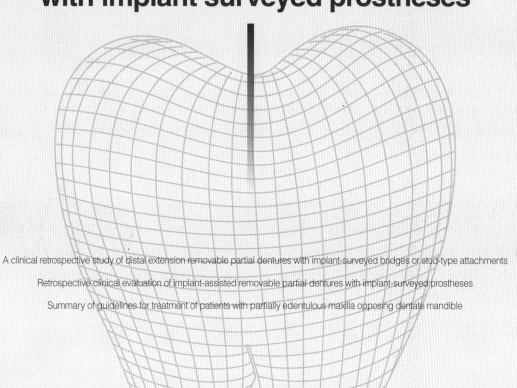

# Representative clinical researches and the summary derived from those studies on IARPD with implant surveyed prostheses

A clinical retrospective study of distal extension removable partial dentures with implant-surveyed bridges or stud-type attachments

Retrospective clinical evaluation of implant-assisted removable partial dentures with implant-surveyed prostheses

Summary of guidelines for treatment of patients with partially edentulous maxilla opposing dentate mandible

*Chapter 5-1.*

# A clinical retrospective study of distal extension removable partial dentures with implant-surveyed bridges or stud-type attachments

This chapter will build upon the content of Chapters 2 and 3 and compare and contrast the results of clinical studies on RPDs using implants as abutments versus RPDs using implant attachments (see Chapter 4.3).

This study was conducted at the Department of Prosthodontics, Pusan National University Dental Hospital to evaluate the efficacy of implant-assisted partial dentures with surveyed bridges through the clinical assessment of implant survival rates and prostheses related complications in two different types of partial denture cases. The first used a surveyed bridge on implants placed in partially edentulous regions as abutments and restored with a distal extension removable partial denture. The second was an overdenture-type removable partial denture made by placing locator attachments on the implants.

## 1. Research subjects

Among the patients treated with implant-assisted removable partial dentures manufactured at the Department of Prosthodontics, Pusan National University Dental Hospital, from 2008 to 2016, those who had been using the dentures for at least one year with regular checkups were included in this study. The participants for this study were selected from the patients who needed implants for additional support and stability in Kennedy class I or II distal extension removable partial dentures, most of whom had mainly complete or partial dentures in their opposing dentition. Patients who had a difference of ten or more degrees between the angle of insertion of the denture and that of implants were excluded from the study. Also, patients with systemic diseases, such as uncontrolled diabetes, cancer, bleeding disorders, immune diseases, or hormonal imbalance, alcohol or drug addiction, and patients who did not attend regular post-treatment check-ups were excluded from the study. A total of 24 patients (6 males, 18 females) who met this criteria were selected for this study after the approval of the Bioethics Committee of the Pusan National University (IRB No. PNUDH- 2015-018).

## 2. Classification of partial dentures

A total of 24 patients were divided into two groups based on the clinical application method used for fabricating the implant-assisted removable partial dentures. The Implant Surveyed Bridge Removable Partial Dentures (ISBRPD) group had conventionally made RPDs with an implant surveyed fixed prosthesis as the abutment. The Implant Attachment Removable Partial Denture (IARPD) group (n = 12) had partial overdentures and locator attachments (Zest Anchors Inc., Escondido, CA, USA) (Figure 1).

## 3. Implant survival rate

In 24 patients with implant-assisted partial dentures, 53 implants were placed: 25 implants in the ISBRPD group and 28 implants in the IARPD group. Of these, 22 implants (ISBRPD group n = 10, IARPD group n = 12) were under functional loads from 12 to 24 months after placement of the partial dentures, and 14 implants were under occlusal load for 25 to 36 months (ISBRPD group n = 8, IARPD group n = 6). There were 17 implants under occlusal load for more than 36 months (ISBRPD n = 7, IARPD n = 10). The mean duration of loading was 26.7 months in the ISBRPD group and 23.5 months in the IARPD group. There were no failed implants and all implants were normal in function without clinical mobility (Table 1).

Table 1. **Cumulative survival rate of the implants.**

| After placement (mo) | ISBRPD group | | | IARPD group | | |
| --- | --- | --- | --- | --- | --- | --- |
| | Implants (N) | Failed implants (N) | CSR (%) | Implants (N) | Failed implants (N) | CSR (%) |
| 12~24 | 10 | - | 100 | 12 | - | 100 |
| 25~36 | 8 | - | 100 | 6 | - | 100 |
| over 36 | 7 | - | 100 | 10 | - | 100 |

CSR: Cumulative survival rate of implants.

## 4. Implant marginal bone resorption and probing depth

The mean values and standard deviations of the implant marginal bone resorption and probing depth are shown in Table 3. The ISBRPD group showed a resorption of 1.44 ± 0.57 mm, a significantly lower implant marginal bone resorption as compared to the IARPD group (p<.05), and there was no significant difference in the probing depth between the two groups (Table 2).

Table 2. **The average value of marginal bone resorption and probing depth.**

|  | ISBRPD group | | IARPD group | | p |
|---|---|---|---|---|---|
|  | Mean | SD | Mean | SD | |
| Marginal bone resorption (mm) | 1.44 | 0.57 | 1.99 | 0.70 | .004* |
| Probing depth (mm) | 3.19 | 0.86 | 3.12 | 0.82 | .817 |

*Mean values showed significant difference based on an independent T-test (p<.05).

## 5. Peri-implant inflammation and bleeding index

In both groups, a normal condition was the most dominantly observed state, and mild inflammation was the next dominant condition observed. Moderate and severe inflammation was not observed. Mild inflammation was not significantly different between the IARPD group (21.4%) and the ISBRPD group (21.7%) (p>.05). Assessment of bleeding index showed that there was no bleeding in the ISBRPD group and the petechia was the most frequent type of bleeding that occurred in the IARPD group. The frequency of petechia bleeding was slightly higher in the IARPD group (39.3%) than in the ISBRPD group (26.1%), but the difference was not significant (p>.05) (Table 3).

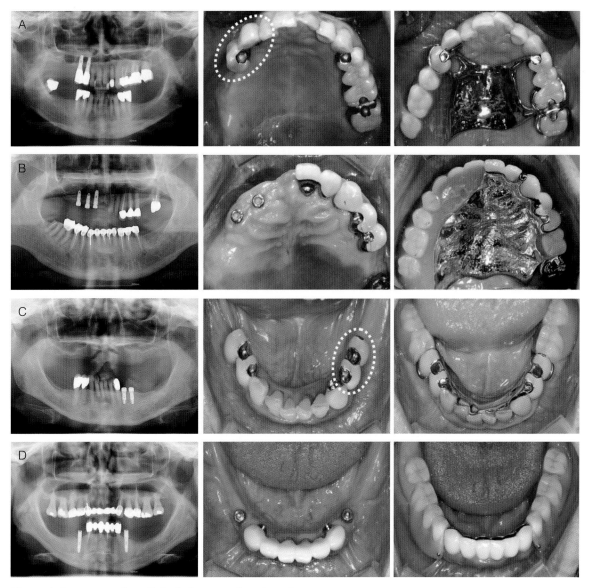

**Figure 1. Representative clinical photographs of study groups.**

(A) ISBRPD group: Fixed surveyed prostheses with two implants (maxillary right canine and first premolar) used as abutments for the RPD.

(B) IARPD group: Locator implant attachments used on top of two implants.

(C) ISBRPD group: Fixed surveyed prostheses with two implants (mandibular left first and second premolar) used as abutments for the RPD.

(D) IARPD group: Locator implant attachments used on top of two implants.

## 6. Plaque index and calculus

No plaque index was observed in the ISBRPD group and a score of 1 was most frequently observed while probing in the IARPD group, but the difference in the plaque index was not significant. The calculus in the ISBRPD group (30.4%) was significantly higher (p<.05) than in the IARPD group (3.6%) (Table 3).

**Table 3. Peri-implant inflammation, bleeding index, plaque index, and calculus.**

|  |  | ISBRPD group† | IARPD group† | p |
|---|---|---|---|---|
| Number of implants |  | 25 | 28 |  |
| Peri-implant inflammation (%) | 0 | 78.3 | 78.6 | 1.000 |
|  | 1 | 21.7 | 21.4 |  |
|  | 2 | - | - |  |
|  | 3 | - | - |  |
| Bleeding index (%) | 0 | 56.5 | 32.1 | .279 |
|  | 1 | 26.1 | 39.3 |  |
|  | 2 | 17.4 | 28.6 |  |
|  | 3 | - | - |  |
| Plaque index (%) | 0 | 47.8 | 28.6 | .121 |
|  | 1 | 21.7 | 50.0 |  |
|  | 2 | 26.1 | 21.4 |  |
|  | 3 | 4.4 | - |  |
| Calculus (%) | 0 | 69.6 | 96.4 | .016* |
|  | 1 | 30.4 | 3.6 |  |

† Frequency distribution of gingival inflammation, bleeding index, plaque index, calculus.

*Frequency distribution showed significant difference based on chi-square test (p<.05).

## 7. Prosthetic complications

Complications occurred more frequently in the IARPD group than in the ISBRPD group. Locator male replacement (64%) and denture repair (22%) were frequent complications in the IARPD group, and denture relining (67%) and denture repair (33%) were frequent complications in the ISBRPD group (Table 4). These complications required maintenance due to the replacement of the locator male in the IARPD group.

Table 4. **Type of clinical complications.**

| | ISBRPD group | IARPD group |
|---|---|---|
| Retention loss | 0 | 14 |
| Screw loosening | 0 | 0 |
| Resin base relining | 4 | 3 |
| Resin base repairing | 2 | 5 |
| Total | 6 | 22 |

## 8. Discussion and conclusion

Long-term clinical studies of removable partial dentures suggest that a stable design and periodic check-ups are important factors affecting the outcome. The use of implant-assisted removable partial dentures with an implant-surveyed bridge or attachments reduces the width of the edentulous area and allows the practitioners to design a more stable removable partial denture.

According to the criteria outlined in Cochran et al.(2002), all implants had a high survival rate, and patients did not experience any mobility and discomfort during the observation period.

The IARPD group showed higher levels of implant marginal bone resorption than the ISBRPD group (p<.05). Adell (1983) reported that marginal bone loss in successful implants disappears after one year of abutment connection, so the prognosis should be assessed after one year. The study conducted by the Brånemark group (1981) reported that one year after the abutment connection was made, marginal bone loss was between 1 and 1.5 mm, with an average of 1.2 mm, and 0.1 mm of marginal bone loss was observed annually thereafter. The average follow-up period was similar in both groups, with 26.7 months in the ISBRPD group and 23.5 months in the IARPD group. It is assumed that the amount of marginal bone resorption is less in the ISBRPD group because the implants are connected by a surveyed bridge, which reduces the stress that causes micro-damage by efficiently dispersing the load generated during mastication.

The two groups showed no significant difference in the plaque index, but the ISBRPD group (p<.05) had a higher calculus index. This result is as expected because it is difficult to maintain oral hygiene due to the characteristics of the fixed prosthesis in ISBRPDs, and it is relatively easier to manage oral hygiene in the IARPD group, which is a solitary type. An implant-surveyed bridge requires a thorough maintenance of oral hygiene, especially on the proximal sides, because it is cemented to the customized abutment which therefore make it more susceptible to acquiring plaque and calculus on the margins of the prosthesis.

Walton et al.(2001) reported that loss of retention in the attachment systems was the most frequently reported complication. Similarly, replacement of the locator attachment occurred most frequently in the lARPD group. On the other hand, the ISBRPD group experienced no loss in retention. The retentive force provided by the clasp can be adjusted relatively easily by the dentist, and if there is no defect in the laboratory process, adjustments are not needed for a relatively long time. However, the maintenance frequency of the locator attachment is high due to wear that results from insertion and dislodgement of the denture, as well as the functional load that is exerted during mastication. Locator attachments are relatively easy to replace and maintain. Other than retention-related complications, there were no other specific complications in the two groups.

In this study, implant marginal bone resorption was significantly higher in the IARPD group than in the ISBRPD group. However, the ISBRPD group showed higher levels of calculus than the IARPD group. Overall clinical complications were more frequent in the IARPD group than in the ISBRPD group. Within the limits of the present study, it was concluded that a well-planned ISBRPD can be clinically appropriate. These results may be a pilot reference point for implant-assisted removable partial dentures using implant-surveyed crowns, and more longitudinal and systematic clinical studies will be necessary to confirm these results.

## REFERENCES

1.  David L. Cochran, Daniel Buser, Christian M. Ten Bruggenkate, Dieter Weingart, Thomas M. Taylor, Jean. Pierre Bernard, Francoise Peters, James P. Simpson. The use of reduced healing times on ITI® implants with a sandblasted and acid.etched (SLA) surface: Early results from clinical trials on ITI® SLA implants. Clin Oral Implants Res 2002; 13:144-53

2.  Adell R. Clinical results of osseointegrated implants supporting fixed prosthesis in edentulous jaw. J Prosthet Dent 1983; 50:251-4.

3.  Adell R, Lekholm U, Rockler B, Brånemark PI. A I5-year study of osseointegrated implants in the treatment of the edentulous jaw. Int J Oral Surg 1981; 10:387-416.

4.  Krennmair G, Krainhofner M, Piehslinger E. Implant-Supported Mandibular Overdentures Retained with a Milled Bar : A Retrospective Study. Int J Oral Maxillofac Implants 2007; 22:987-94.

5.  Lindquist LW, Rockier B, Carlsson GE. Bone resorption around fixtures in edentulous patients treated with mandibular fixed tissue-integrated prostheses. J Prosthet Dent 1988; 59:63.

6.  Walton JN, Huizinga SC, Peck CC. Implant angulation: A measurement technique, implant overdenture maintenance, and the influence of surgical experience. Int J Prosthodont 2001; 14:523-30.

7.  Payne AG, Tawse.Smith A, Wismeijer D, De Silva RK, Ma S. Multicentre prospective evaluation of implant.assisted mandibular removable partial dentures: surgical and prosthodontic outcomes. Clin Oral Implants Res 2017; 28:116-25.

8.  Bae EB, Kim SJ, Choi JW, Jeon YC, Jeong CM, Yun MJ, Lee SH, Huh JB. A Clinical Retrospective Study of Distal Extension Removable Partial Denture with Implant Surveyed Bridge or Stud Type Attachment. Biomed Res Int. 2017;2017:7140870.

# Chapter 5-2.

# Retrospective clinical evaluation of implant-assisted removable partial dentures with implant-surveyed prostheses

This chapter will build upon the content from Chapters 2 and 3, and further, compare clinical studies of RPDs that use implants as abutments (Chapter 4.2). Implant-assisted removable partial dentures have been suggested as an alternative treatment option for partial edentulism. However, evidence supporting the efficacy of IARPDs combined with implant surveyed prostheses as abutments is limited. The following study, however, outlines how IARPDs using implant surveyed prostheses could be a viable treatment option for partial edentulism.

In previous studies, implant-surveyed prostheses showed less marginal bone resorption and loss of retention than attachments did, possibly due to more frequent maintenance and fewer prosthetic-related complications. Though IARPDs using implant-surveyed prostheses are a potential treatment option, there are still a limited number of studies available to support their use.

Therefore, the purpose of this study was to evaluate the clinical status of IARPDs using implant-surveyed prostheses with respect to clinical tissue conditions, marginal bone resorption, and prosthetic complications. The study hoped to show that implant-surveyed prostheses can be successfully implemented as abutments for IARPDs.

## 1. Research subjects

This retrospective clinical study was conducted on patients wearing IARPDs with implant-surveyed prostheses as abutments (IRB number: PNUDH-2015-018).

All patients had worn their dentures for at least 12 months and received regular maintenance check-ups. Based on the study by Chikunov et al.(2008), partially edentulous patients requiring dental implants for additional retention, support, and stability of RPDs were selected. Patients who had suffered from alveolar bone resorption resulting in an insufficient number of implants and patients who needed a denture providing soft tissue support were included. Additionally, patients who were unable to undergo invasive surgery because of systemic diseases, age, or other reasons were included.

Patients with a history of uncontrolled diabetes mellitus, cardiovascular disease, or alcoholism, those that had received radiotherapy in the head and neck region for malignancy, and those with severe temporomandibular joint disorders were excluded.

A total of 24 participants (21 women, 3 men) were selected for the study. The mean age was 67.5 years and the average follow-up period was 27.6 months (maximum 78 months) (Table 1). During the initial visit, chief complaints and medical history were recorded, and oral hygiene management ability and patient expectations were evaluated. Clinical and radiological examinations were performed to evaluate the state of the remaining teeth, the position and size of edentulous sites, and the residual alveolar bone quality. The state of the opposing dentition, flatness of the occlusal plane, and occlusal relations were also evaluated.

Table 1. **Data on patients and implants.**

| Patient | Gender | Age (y) | Restored arch | Kennedy class | Type of opposing dentition | Number of RPD abutments (implant) | Number of RPD abutments (natural teeth) | Follow-up period (months) |
|---|---|---|---|---|---|---|---|---|
| 1 | M | 70 | Mn | I | C | 5 | 0 | 12 |
| 2 | F | 53 | Mx | IV | F | 7 | 2 | 13 |
| 3 | F | 71 | Mn | I | R | 2 | 4 | 20 |
| 4 | F | 73 | Mx | I | R | 2 | 4 | 42 |
| | | | Mn | I | R | 4 | 4 | 26 |
| 5 | F | 67 | Mx | I | R | 5 | 2 | 13 |
| 6 | F | 76 | MX | I | F | 4 | 4 | 72 |
| 7 | F | 73 | MX | I | R | 2 | 4 | 78 |
| 8 | F | 67 | Mn | I | C | 2 | 2 | 60 |
| 9 | F | 66 | Mn | I | R | 4 | 0 | 59 |
| 10 | M | 46 | Mn | I | F | 3 | 0 | 42 |
| 11 | F | 64 | Mn | I | C | 3 | 1 | 13 |
| 12 | F | 60 | Mn | I | F | 1 | 3 | 12 |
| 13 | F | 71 | Mx | II | C | 2 | 4 | 14 |
| 14 | F | 71 | Mx | I | F | 4 | 0 | 13 |
| 15 | F | 71 | Mn | I | R | 2 | 1 | 12 |
| 16 | F | 69 | Mn | I | R | 2 | 5 | 22 |
| 17 | F | 61 | Mx | II | F | 2 | 3 | 15 |
| 18 | F | 54 | Mx | I | F | 1 | 4 | 15 |
| 19 | F | 67 | Mx | IV | R | 2 | 0 | 12 |
| 20 | F | 75 | Mn | II | F | 3 | 2 | 13 |

| 21 | F | 71 | Mx | I | F | 2 | 4 | 69 |
| 22 | M | 71 | Mx | IV | F | 5 | 2 | 15 |
| 23 | F | 72 | Mx | IV | F | 6 | 2 | 15 |
| 24 | F | 80 | Mn | I | C | 5 | 0 | 13 |

*Types of opposing dentition: F, natural dentition and fixed prosthesis; R, removable partial denture; C, complete denture.

Treatment plans were established after diagnosis, and all treatments were performed with patient consent. Teeth with poor prognosis were extracted, and restorative and periodontal treatments were performed on residual teeth. Provisional prostheses were then fabricated and delivered for occlusal supports.

A dental CT was used to evaluate residual bone quality for implant placement. When only anterior teeth were remaining, implant placement was planned for the anterior region with sufficient bone volume (height > 8 mm and diameter > 3.5 mm) for IARPDs with a short edentulous area. Placing of implants adjacent to the residual teeth enabled better stress distribution in teeth and supporting tissues. Based on the consideration of the RPD abutment symmetry in the same arch, implants were placed in positions where occlusion would be with opposing natural or implant teeth.

After the healing period, surveyed fixed prostheses were made for residual teeth and implants were used as abutments. The contours of the implant surveyed prostheses were consistent with the RPD insertion. The buccal surfaces of the implant-surveyed prostheses were fabricated to provide proper retention. Besides, retainers were designed to accommodate for potential denture movements, occlusal rests had adequate length and thickness, and major connectors had sufficient strength. Functional impressions were taken and altered casts were fabricated to obtain support for the distal extension bases. This minimized the lateral forces exerted on the implant abutments.

The artificial teeth of the RPDs had definite occlusal contact to ensure that excessive force was not applied to the implants. In addition, participants were thoroughly educated about oral hygiene management, the necessity of wearing dentures during meals, and denture cleaning. Figure 1 shows an example of this treatment method.

Regular check-ups were performed one day, one week, and one month post-denture delivery and regular follow-ups were performed every six months thereafter.

During the last regular follow-up, clinical and radiological examinations were conducted.

In this study, we evaluated the clinical applicability of using IARPDs with implant-surveyed prostheses. To evaluate implant abutments, we examined implant survival rates, marginal bone resorption, probing depths, calculus, peri-inflammation, bleeding, and plaque indices, which have long been widely used to evaluate implants in implant fixed prostheses.

## 2. Results from this study

A total of 24 participants and 25 prostheses (12 maxilla and 13 mandible prostheses) were analyzed. In one participant, both the maxilla and the mandible were treated with IARPDs using implant-surveyed prostheses. According to the Kennedy classification, 18 prostheses were Class I, three were Class II, and four were of Class IV. None of the Class III patients were treated. Regarding the opposing dentition, ten prostheses had natural dentition or fixed prostheses, nine prostheses had a removable partial denture, and five prostheses had a complete denture.

A total of 80 implants were used as abutments for IARPDs. The distribution of implants is shown in Table 2. In the maxilla, implants were mostly placed in the premolar area. In the mandible, the implants were placed mostly in the canine and premolar areas. 78 implants were splinted, and two were restored with a single implant surveyed prosthesis.

**Table 2. Distributions of implants. (n)**

|     | Incisor | Canine | Premolar | Molar |
|-----|---------|--------|----------|-------|
| Mx  | 4       | 6      | 21       | 13    |
| Mn  | 8       | 12     | 15       | 1     |

An analysis of the role of implant surveyed prostheses in IARPDs, showed that 40 implants (50%) provided retention, whereas 28 implants (35%) provided support. 12 implants (15%) were used for stabilization and abutment strengthening. The direct retainers used were RPA, RPI, Akers, or embrasure clasps, but RPAs were most frequently used. Monolithic zirconia was the most commonly used material for implant surveyed prostheses. Other materials included porcelain-fused-to-metal (PFM, 27 implants), porcelain-fused-to-gold (PFG, 12 implants), and porcelain-fused-to-innovium (PFI, 6 implants).

Table 3 shows implant numbers and cumulative survival rates. All the examined implants were functioning normally without any signs of mobility. The mean marginal bone resorption of implants one year after loading was $0.772 \pm 0.63$ mm (Table 4). Material, restored arch, design, and opposing dentition were not found to significantly influence marginal bone resorption. The overall mean probing depth was $3.36 \pm 0.06$ mm (Table 4) and the mean probing depth for maxillary implants was significantly greater than that of mandibular implants ($p=.007$). Table 5 shows the results of the peri-implant inflammation index. A score 0 (73.01%) inflammation was the most common score in the peri-implant inflammation index, and a score of 1 (26.98%) was reported. Scores 2 and 3 were not observed. Peri-implant inflammation index ratios were not influenced by subgroups. In terms of the gingival bleeding index, a score of 0 (42.85%), indicating no bleeding, was dominant. A score of

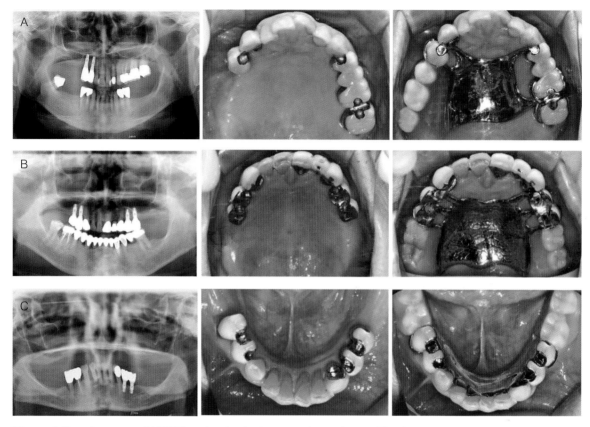

**Figure 1.** Sample cases of IARPDs using implant surveyed prostheses. Fixed surveyed prostheses with (A) two implants (maxillary right canine and first premolar), (B) four implants (maxillary bilateral first and second premolar), and (C) two implants (mandibular left first and second premolar) used as abutments for the RPD.

1 was 30.15%, a score of 2 was 25.39%, and a score of 3 was 1.59% of all reported scores. There was no significant difference between subgroups (Table 6). A score of 0 (68.25%), indicating no plaque, was observed most frequently, compared to scores of 1 (14.28%) and 2 (17.46%). A score of 3 was not observed. No significant difference was observed between subgroups (Table 7). No calculus was detected on any of the implant abutments.

**Table 3. Cumulative survival rates of the implants.**

| Months after placement | Implants (n) | Failed implants (n) | Cumulative survival rate (%) |
|:---:|:---:|:---:|:---:|
| 0-12 | 10 | - | 100 |
| 13-24 | 47 | - | 100 |
| 25-36 | 3 | - | 100 |
| 37-48 | 5 | - | 100 |
| Over 48 | 14 | - | 100 |

**Table 4. Mean marginal bone resorptions and probing depths. (mm)**

| | | Marginal bone resorption | | | Probing depth | | |
|---|---|---|---|---|---|---|---|
| Total | | Mean | SD | p | Mean | SD | p |
| | | 0.772 | 0.63 | | 3.36 | 0.06 | |
| Materials | PFM | 0.736 | 0.67 | >.05 | 3.48 | 0.80 | >.05 |
| | MZ | 0.795 | 0.61 | | 3.19 | 0.49 | |
| Site | Mx | 0.821 | 0.65 | >.05 | 3.51 | 0.65 | .007 |
| | Mn | 0.616 | 0.55 | | 3.05 | 0.56 | |
| Design | Retention | 0.777 | 0.67 | >.05 | 3.32 | 0.71 | >.05 |
| | Support | 0.579 | 0.43 | | 3.12 | 0.47 | |
| Opposing dentition | F | 0.672 | 0.16 | | 3.51 | 0.73 | |
| | R | 0.905 | 0.16 | >.05 | 3.29 | 0.54 | >.05 |
| | C | 0.999 | 0.61 | | 3.00 | 0.61 | |

Whether the difference in mean values were significant was calculated using an independent T-test (p<.05).

*Materials: PFM, porcelain fused to metal; MZ, monolithic zirconia

*Opposing dentition: F, natural dentition and fixed prosthesis; R, removable partial denture; C, complete denture.

**Table 5. Peri-implant inflammation scores. (%)**

| | | Score 0 | Score 1 | Score 2 | Score 3 | p |
|---|---|---|---|---|---|---|
| Total | | 73.01 | 26.98 | 0 | 0 | |
| Materials | PFM | 73.91 | 26.08 | 0 | 0 | >.05 |
| | MZ | 73.91 | 26.08 | 0 | 0 | |
| Site | Mx | 71.42 | 28.57 | 0 | 0 | >.05 |
| | Mn | 72.72 | 27.27 | 0 | 0 | |
| Design | Retention | 75.00 | 25.00 | 0 | 0 | >.05 |
| | Support | 44.83 | 35.00 | 0 | 0 | |
| Opposing dentition | F | 77.41 | 22.58 | 0 | 0 | |
| | R | 66.67 | 33.33 | 0 | 0 | >.05 |
| | C | 66.67 | 33.33 | 0 | 0 | |

*Materials: PFM, porcelain fused to metal; MZ, monolithic zirconia

*Opposing dentition: F, natural dentition and fixed prosthesis; R, removable partial denture; C, complete denture.

Table 6. **Bleeding index scores. (%)**

| Total | | Score 0<br>42.85 | Score 1<br>30.15 | Score 2<br>25.39 | Score 3<br>1.59 | p |
|---|---|---|---|---|---|---|
| Materials | PFM | 21.74 | 43.48 | 34.78 | 0 | >.05 |
| | Zirconia | 47.82 | 30.43 | 21.74 | 0 | |
| Site | Mx | 38.10 | 38.10 | 26.19 | 2.38 | >.05 |
| | Mn | 54.54 | 13.64 | 31.82 | 0 | |
| Design | Retention | 37.50 | 40.62 | 18.75 | 3.12 | >.05 |
| | Support | 50.00 | 10.00 | 40.00 | 0 | |
| Opposing dentition | F | 48.39 | 32.26 | 16.13 | 3.22 | |
| | R | 20.83 | 37.50 | 41.67 | 0 | >.05 |
| | C | 66.67 | 0 | 33.33 | 0 | |

*Materials: PFM, porcelain fused to metal; MZ, monolithic zirconia

*Opposing dentition: F, natural dentition and fixed prosthesis; R, removable partial denture; C, complete denture

Table 7. **Plaque index scores. (%)**

| Total | | Score 0<br>68.25 | Score 1<br>14.28 | Score 2<br>17.46 | Score 3<br>0 | p |
|---|---|---|---|---|---|---|
| Materials | PFM | 60.87 | 17.39 | 21.73 | 0 | >.05 |
| | Zirconia | 78.26 | 21.74 | 0 | 0 | |
| Site | Mx | 64.28 | 21.43 | 14.28 | 0 | >.05 |
| | Mn | 72.73 | 4.54 | 22.73 | 0 | |
| Design | Retention | 71.87 | 9.37 | 18.75 | 0 | >.05 |
| | Support | 65.00 | 15.00 | 20.00 | 0 | |
| Opposing dentition | F | 70.97 | 16.13 | 12.90 | 0 | |
| | R | 66.67 | 8.33 | 25.00 | 0 | >.05 |
| | C | 55.55 | 33.33 | 11.11 | 0 | |

*Materials: PFM, porcelain fused to metal; MZ, monolithic zirconia

*Opposing dentition: F, natural dentition and fixed prosthesis; R, removable partial denture; C, complete denture

In terms of denture-related complications, two clasp fractures occurred in one patient and one rest fracture occurred in another. In terms of implant-surveyed prosthesis-related complications, one patient treated with a cement-retained implant fixed prosthesis required re-cementation of the prosthesis, and another patient showed marginal bone resorption due to excess cement. A porcelain fracture in a PFM implant surveyed prosthesis occurred in one patient.

## 3. Conclusion from this study

Using implant-surveyed prostheses as abutments for IARPDs yielded favorable results. IARPDs combined with implant surveyed prostheses enhance retention, support, and stability in partially edentulous patients. However, proper case selection, implant placements, and denture designs are essential. Further long-term clinical evaluations are also necessary to ensure the reliability of this treatment method.

## REFERENCES

1. Bae EB, Kim SJ, Choi JW, Jeon YC, Jeong CM, Yun MJ, Lee SH, Huh JB. A Clinical Retrospective Study of Distal Extension Removable Partial Denture with Implant Surveyed Bridge or Stud Type Attachment. Biomed Res Int 2017; 2017:1-7.

2. Chikunov I, Doan P, Vahidi F. Implant-retained partial overdenture with resilient attachments. J Prosthodont 2008; 17:141-8.

3. Keltjens HM, Kayser AF, Hertel R, Battistuzzi PG. Distal extension removable partial dentures supported by implants and residual teeth: considerations and case reports. Int J Oral Maxillofac Implants 1993; 8:208-13.

4. Wismeijer D, Tawse-Smith A, Payne AG. Multicentre prospective evaluation of implant-assisted mandibular bilateral distal extension removable partial dentures: Patient satisfaction. Clin Oral Implants 2013; 24:20-2.

5. Cunha LD, Pellizzer EP, Verri FR, Pereira JA. Evaluation of the influence of location of osseointegrated implants associated with mandibular removable partial dentures. Implant Dent 2008; 17:278-87.

6. Park JM, Koak JY, Kim SK, Joo JH, Heo SJ. Consideration for the Combination Treatment of Removable Partial Denture and Implant. Implantol 2015; 19:104-11.

7. Shahmiri R, Das R, Aarts JM, Bennani V. Finite element analysis of an implant-assisted removable partial denture during bilateral loading: Occlusal rests position. J Prosthet Dent 2014; 112:1126-33.

8. Shahmiri R, Das R. Finite element analysis of implant-assisted removable partial dentures: Framework design considerations. J Prosthet Dent 2017; 118:177-86.

9. Lee YJ, Bae EB, Jeong CM, Lee JJ, Kim JY, Huh JB. Removable Partial Denture Using Anterior Implant-Supported Fixed Prostheses for Edentulous Patients. J Korean Dent Sci 2017; 10:87-95.

10. Papaspyridakos P, Chen CJ, Singh M, Weber HP, Gallucci GO. Success criteria in implant dentistry: a systematic review. J Dent Res 2012; 91:242-8.

11. Albrektsson T, Zarb G, Worthington P, Eriksson AR. The long-term efficacy of currently used dental implants: a review and proposed criteria of success. Int J Oral Maxillofac Implants 1986; 1:11-25.

12. Oh YK, Bae EB, Huh JB. Retrospective clinical evaluation of implant-assisted removable partial dentures combined with implant surveyed prostheses. J Prosthet Dent. 2020 Aug 10;S0022-3913(20)30297-3. Online ahead of print.

Chapter 5-3.

# Summary of guidelines for treatment of patients with partially edentulous maxilla opposing dentate mandible

After giving careful consideration to the entire gamut of implant-assisted RPDs, I have concluded that it is difficult to suggest precise treatment guidelines since there are a wide variety of clinical cases, and having a thorough understanding of the basic RPD concepts is important to establish a treatment plan.

For this reason, a more profound discussion about the design of metal framework, impression, occlusion and maintenance is given in this book. A firm grounding in the basics would make complex removable partial denture cases much easier to deal with and patient comfort would be improved by placing additional implants.

I would like to emphasize to my readers that prosthodontic treatment, especially removable partial denture treatment, should abide by the basic knowledge of partial dentures; and precise decision making and abundant experience of the dentist are important since there are a wide range of cases of removable partial dentures that may be presented. There are schools of thought that implants are placed to change tooth and tissue-supported RPDs into tooth-supported RPDs. Is that really true? However, the overriding principle is that implant placement and dental prostheses selection must be conducted in a way to ensure that the occlusion force is distributed in the most stable manner by investigating the opposing teeth, occlusal force and patterns, and the status of the tissue support area.

I hope that this book would be of assistance to clinicians in the treatment of implant-assisted RPD.

The following table is a summary of guidelines assuming that patients with partially edentulous maxilla opposing dentate mandible are given an option of placing only two additional implants in the maxilla. This table is highly subjective and does not offer an exact right answer; there may exist many other diverse solutions as well. I would like to conclude this book by sharing some points to consider in the course of treatment planning.

| Maxilla | Location of implants | Implant prostheses | Advantages | Disadvantages |
|---|---|---|---|---|
| | | Left maxillary 1$^{st}$ and 2$^{nd}$ premolar surveyed bridge | 1. Splinting<br>2. Aesthetic when not wearing the RPD<br>3. Ease of the RPD design due to symmetry of remaining teeth<br>4. Sufficient support, stability and retention<br>5. Ease of maintenance and repair through conventional RPD fabrication | 1. Lack of support in both maxillary posterior areas<br>2. Exposure of clasps |
| | | Left maxillary 1$^{st}$ premolar and 2$^{nd}$ molar surveyed bridge | 1. Aesthetic when wearing RPD<br>2. Stable posterior occlusal support on the left | 1. Fabrication of RPD needed for restoration of the right molar area<br>2. Excessive occlusal force on 4-unit bridge supported by two implants<br>3. Excessive lateral force on the implants from RPD movement |
| | | Left 1$^{st}$ premolar and right 1$^{st}$ molar attachments (assuming the use of locator attachments) | 1. Additional support and stability along with retention when a locator is used (differs depending on the type of attachments used)<br>2. Removal of clasp is possible since retention can be obtained from attachments | 1. Limitations in design due to bilateral asymmetry<br>2. For long-term use of attachments, design minor connectors that give enough stability and place implants parallel to the path of insertion of RPD<br>3. Splinting is not possible<br>4. Maintenance of the overdenture is necessary due to the wear of attachments |

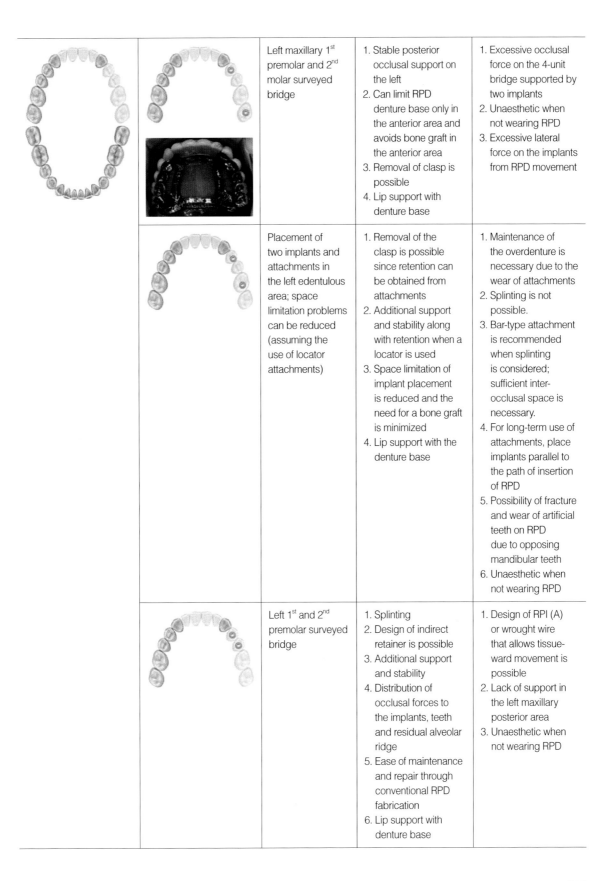

| | | Left maxillary 1st premolar and 2nd molar surveyed bridge | 1. Stable posterior occlusal support on the left<br>2. Can limit RPD denture base only in the anterior area and avoids bone graft in the anterior area<br>3. Removal of clasp is possible<br>4. Lip support with denture base | 1. Excessive occlusal force on the 4-unit bridge supported by two implants<br>2. Unaesthetic when not wearing RPD<br>3. Excessive lateral force on the implants from RPD movement |
|---|---|---|---|---|
| | | Placement of two implants and attachments in the left edentulous area; space limitation problems can be reduced (assuming the use of locator attachments) | 1. Removal of the clasp is possible since retention can be obtained from attachments<br>2. Additional support and stability along with retention when a locator is used<br>3. Space limitation of implant placement is reduced and the need for a bone graft is minimized<br>4. Lip support with the denture base | 1. Maintenance of the overdenture is necessary due to the wear of attachments<br>2. Splinting is not possible.<br>3. Bar-type attachment is recommended when splinting is considered; sufficient inter-occlusal space is necessary.<br>4. For long-term use of attachments, place implants parallel to the path of insertion of RPD<br>5. Possibility of fracture and wear of artificial teeth on RPD due to opposing mandibular teeth<br>6. Unaesthetic when not wearing RPD |
| | | Left 1st and 2nd premolar surveyed bridge | 1. Splinting<br>2. Design of indirect retainer is possible<br>3. Additional support and stability<br>4. Distribution of occlusal forces to the implants, teeth and residual alveolar ridge<br>5. Ease of maintenance and repair through conventional RPD fabrication<br>6. Lip support with denture base | 1. Design of RPI (A) or wrought wire that allows tissue-ward movement is possible<br>2. Lack of support in the left maxillary posterior area<br>3. Unaesthetic when not wearing RPD |

| | | Left and right lateral incisors implant bridge | 1. Aesthetic when not wearing RPD<br>2. Additional support is obtained in the anterior maxilla | 1. Bone graft might be necessary in the anterior area of the maxilla<br>2. Difficulty in design due to unilaterally edentulous posterior area<br>3. Design of stress breaker type direct retainer and indirect retainer in tooth and tissue supported RPD is important<br>4. Stability is established through functional impression and occlusal scheme<br>5. Lack of support in the left maxillary posterior area<br>6. Exposure of clasp in the anterior maxilla |
| | | Left canine and 1st premolar surveyed bridge | 1. Aesthetic when not wearing RPD<br>2. Increased support and stability in the anterior region through additional rests and minor connector<br>3. Ease of design of RPI or RPA on the 1st premolar<br>4. Ease of applying support and indirect retention on the right remaining teeth<br>5. Splinting | 1. Impression taking of the edentulous area is still important for tooth and tissue supported RPDs even if the edentulous area is shortened<br>2. Need a design that gives maximum stability to the remaining abutment teeth and prevents lateral force to the implants<br>3. Extension of the implant support area and easier RPD treatment become possible if a 3-unit implant surveyed bridge is fabricated on the left canine and 1st premolar |

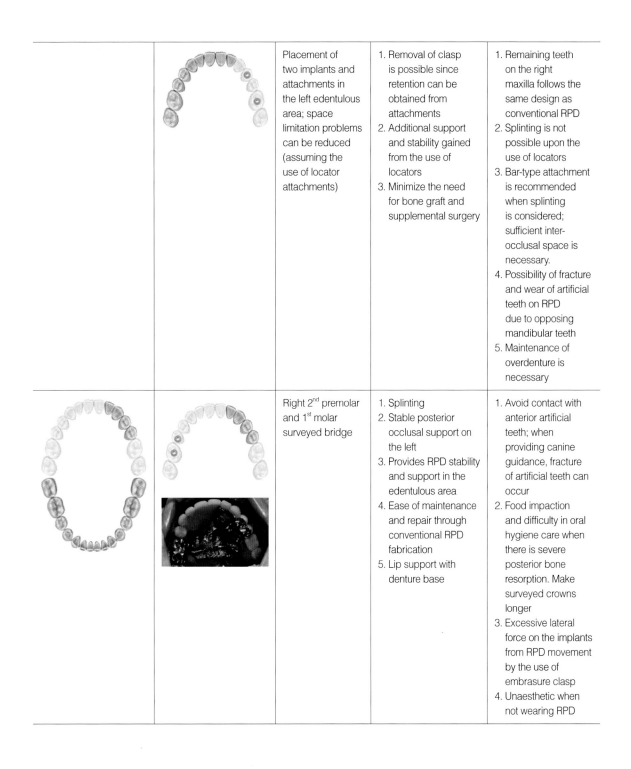

| | | Placement of two implants and attachments in the left edentulous area; space limitation problems can be reduced (assuming the use of locator attachments) | 1. Removal of clasp is possible since retention can be obtained from attachments<br>2. Additional support and stability gained from the use of locators<br>3. Minimize the need for bone graft and supplemental surgery | 1. Remaining teeth on the right maxilla follows the same design as conventional RPD<br>2. Splinting is not possible upon the use of locators<br>3. Bar-type attachment is recommended when splinting is considered; sufficient inter-occlusal space is necessary.<br>4. Possibility of fracture and wear of artificial teeth on RPD due to opposing mandibular teeth<br>5. Maintenance of overdenture is necessary |
| | | Right 2nd premolar and 1st molar surveyed bridge | 1. Splinting<br>2. Stable posterior occlusal support on the left<br>3. Provides RPD stability and support in the edentulous area<br>4. Ease of maintenance and repair through conventional RPD fabrication<br>5. Lip support with denture base | 1. Avoid contact with anterior artificial teeth; when providing canine guidance, fracture of artificial teeth can occur<br>2. Food impaction and difficulty in oral hygiene care when there is severe posterior bone resorption. Make surveyed crowns longer<br>3. Excessive lateral force on the implants from RPD movement by the use of embrasure clasp<br>4. Unaesthetic when not wearing RPD |

| | | | | |
|---|---|---|---|---|
| | | Left incisor and right canine surveyed bridge | 1. Aesthetic when wearing RPD<br>2. Additional support is obtained in the anterior maxilla<br>3. Design of indirect retainer is possible when rest seat is formed | 1. Movement of RPD exists due to the long edentulous area (unstable RPD)<br>2. Wrought wire on the right canine is recommended<br>3. Lack of support and stability in both maxillary posterior areas<br>4. Bone graft might be necessary in the anterior area of the maxilla<br>5. Lack of lip support |
| | | Right canine and 2nd premolar 3-unit surveyed bridge | 1. Splinting<br>2. Ease of design due to symmetry of posterior edentulous region<br>3. Distribution of occlusal forces to the implants, teeth, and residual alveolar ridge<br>4. Lip support with denture base | 1. Unaesthetic when not wearing RPD<br>2. Functional impression of the posterior area is still needed<br>3. Excessive lateral force on the implants from RPD movement |
| | | Right lateral incisor and 1st premolar 3-unit surveyed bridge | 1. Aesthetic when wearing RPD<br>2. Additional support is obtained in the anterior maxilla<br>3. Placing direct retainer, acting as stress breaker on the right 2nd premolar is possible | 1. Movement of RPD exists due to the long edentulous area (unstable RPD)<br>2. Possibility of RPD fracture and abutment damage due to long span edentulous area in the left<br>3. Insufficient stability due to low number of remaining teeth<br>4. Excessive lateral force on the implants from RPD movement |

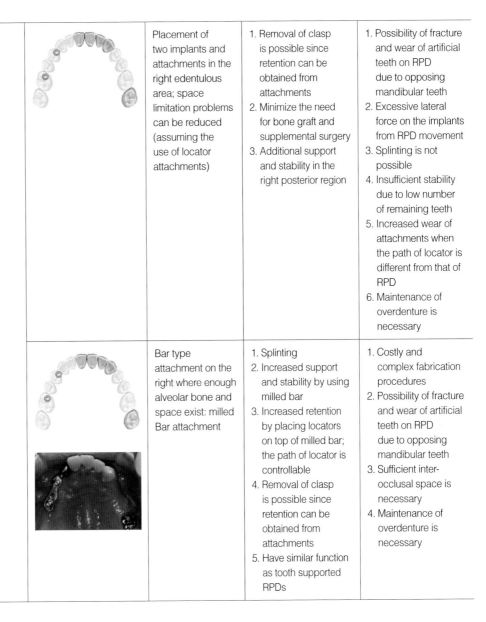

| | Placement of two implants and attachments in the right edentulous area; space limitation problems can be reduced (assuming the use of locator attachments) | 1. Removal of clasp is possible since retention can be obtained from attachments<br>2. Minimize the need for bone graft and supplemental surgery<br>3. Additional support and stability in the right posterior region | 1. Possibility of fracture and wear of artificial teeth on RPD due to opposing mandibular teeth<br>2. Excessive lateral force on the implants from RPD movement<br>3. Splinting is not possible<br>4. Insufficient stability due to low number of remaining teeth<br>5. Increased wear of attachments when the path of locator is different from that of RPD<br>6. Maintenance of overdenture is necessary |
| | Bar type attachment on the right where enough alveolar bone and space exist: milled Bar attachment | 1. Splinting<br>2. Increased support and stability by using milled bar<br>3. Increased retention by placing locators on top of milled bar; the path of locator is controllable<br>4. Removal of clasp is possible since retention can be obtained from attachments<br>5. Have similar function as tooth supported RPDs | 1. Costly and complex fabrication procedures<br>2. Possibility of fracture and wear of artificial teeth on RPD due to opposing mandibular teeth<br>3. Sufficient inter-occlusal space is necessary<br>4. Maintenance of overdenture is necessary |

**Thank you for providing clinical cases in addition to your guidance and support with expertise in the field of Prosthodontics.**

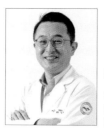

Chang Mo Jeong

Professor
School of Dentistry
Pusan National University

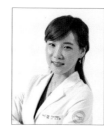

So Hyoun Lee

Associate Professor
School of Dentistry
Pusan National University

**Thank you for being great clinical assistants during your residency training period, and helping out in various ways to make the publication of this book possible.**

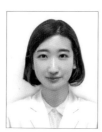

You Kyoung Oh

Bachelor of Science in Dental Laboratory, Korea University
DDS, School of Dentistry, Pusan National University
Prosthodontist, Department of Prosthodontics, Pusan National University Dental Hospital

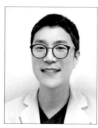

Jin Wan Kim

Bachelor of Science in Biotechnology, Yonsei University
DDS, School of Dentistry, Pusan National University
Prosthodontist, Department of Prosthodontics, Pusan National University Dental Hospital

**Thank you for your meticulous efforts in guiding me through the translation process of this book.**

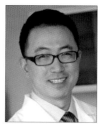

Joo H Kwon

University of Illinois, College of Dentistry
Dio Implant Key Doctor/Instructor
Private Practice in Round Lake Beach and Waukegan, IL

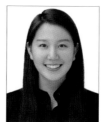

Janet Lee

Bachelor of Arts in Psychology, University of Pennsylvania class of 2022

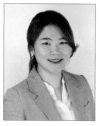

Ja Young Lee

Bachelor of Science in Biochemistry, McGill University
DDS, School of Dentistry, Pusan National University

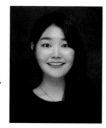

Ju Young Lee

Bachelor of Arts & Science in Biology, McGill University
DDS, School of Dentistry, Pusan National University

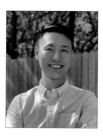

Joung Lee

Bachelor of Science in biochemistry from Georgia Tech
DDS, Nova Southeastern University School of Dental Medicine in Florida with oral surgery honor

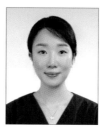

Soyun Kim

Bachelor of Science in Biochemistry and Cell Biology, University of California, San Diego
DDS, School of Dentistry, Pusan National University
Prosthodontic Residency program, Department of Prosthodontics, University of Pennsylvania

**Thank you for sharing your talent in creating user-friendly illustrations for better understanding.**

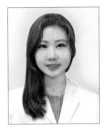

Eun Bin Bae

Ph.D. Department of Prosthodontics,
Pusan National University

**I would also like to thank my dear students who put in a great deal of effort into learning about IARPD and making this publication. I hope it will be of help in their future.**

**[ PNU IARPD Research group ]**

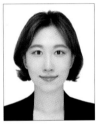

Joon Hee Park

Bachelor of Science in Biomedical
Engineering, Hanyang University
DDS, School of Dentistry, Pusan
National University
Prosthodontist, Department of Prost-
hodontics, Ewha Womans University
Mokdong Hospital.

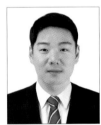

Sang Woo Kim

Bachelor of Science in Biology,
University of California San Diego
DDS, School of Dentistry, Pusan
National Universityal

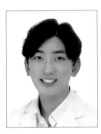

Sae Woong Hyun

Bachelor of Science in Biology,
University of Kentucky
DDS, School of Dentistry, Pusan
National University

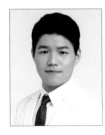

Sung Ha Park

Bachelor of Science in Biochemistry,
University of Bath
DDS, School of Dentistry, Pusan
National University

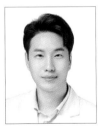

Jae Young Ahn

Bachelor of Science in Chemistry,
University of Southern California
DDS, School of Dentistry, Pusan
National University

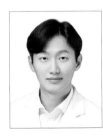

Jae Woo Nam

Bachelor of Science in Biochemistry,
Hong Kong University of Science
and Technology
DDS, School of Dentistry, Pusan
National University

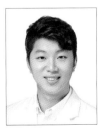

Jeung Ho Lee

Bachelor of Science in General
Biology, University of California
San Diego
DDS, School of Dentistry, Pusan
National University

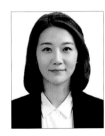

Min Jung Kim

Bachelor of Science in Biology, Pusan
National University
DDS, School of Dentistry, Pusan National
University
Prosthodontist, Department of Prosthodontics,
Pusan National University Dental Hospital